Access to Anaesthetics Primary FRCA Pocket Book 2: Physics, Clinical Measurement and Equipment MCQs

Kirsty MacLennan MBChB, MRCP, FRCA

Specialist Registrar Anaesthesia

North West Region

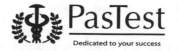
Dedicated to your success

First Published 2007

ISBN: 1905 635 303
ISBN: 978 1905 635 306

A catalogue record for this book is available from the British Library.

The information contained within this book was obtained by the author from reliable sources. However, while every effort has been made to ensure its accuracy, no responsibility for loss, damage or injury occasioned to any person acting or refraining from action as a result of information contained herein can be accepted by the publishers or author.

PasTest Revision Books and Intensive Courses

PasTest has been established in the field of postgraduate medical education since 1972, providing revision books and intensive study courses for doctors preparing for their professional examinations.

Books and courses are available for the following specialties:
MRCGP, MRCP Parts 1 and 2, MRCPCH Parts 1 and 2, MRCPsych, MRCS, MRCOG Parts 1 and 2, DRCOG, DCH, FRCA, PLAB Parts 1 and 2.

For further details contact:
PasTest, Freepost, Knutsford, Cheshire WA16 7BR
Tel: 01565 752000 Fax: 01565 650264
www.pastest.co.uk enquiries@pastest.co.uk

Typeset by Keytec Typesetting Ltd, Bridport, Dorset, UK
Printed and bound in the UK by Athenaeum Press, Gateshead.

CONTENTS

CONTENTS

ACKNOWLEDGEMENTS

I would like to thank Dr. Nolan for taking the time to write the foreword; Dr. Whitaker for his review; Dr. S. Maguire, Dr. K. Grady and Dr. W. de Mello for their advice and encouragement.

I would also like to thank the publishers, PasTest, my family, who have supported me. And above all, Ann MacLennan who has been my rock as always!

FOREWORD

The introduction of run-through training in Anaesthesia and the need for the Royal College of Anaesthetists [RCOA] to structure timing and content of Postgraduate examinations in accordance with the requirements of the Postgraduate Medical and Education Training Board [PMETB] has led to recent changes to the Primary Fellowship of the Royal College of Anaesthetists [FRCA] examination.

The Primary Multiple Choice Question [MCQ] examination became a "stand alone" Pass/Fail examination in June 2007. A close marking scheme is used where 1 is a poor fail, 1+ is a fail, 2 is a Pass and a 2+ reflects an outstanding performance. The Primary FRCA MCQ examination consists of 90 questions undertaken in three hours and comprises three subsections of 30 MCQs examining Pharmacology, Physiology, Physics and Clinical Measurement. A mark of 2 is required to pass the MCQ although a candidate who significantly underperforms in one or more subsection of the MCQ will fail the examination. Negative marking is applied with one mark being deducted for each incorrect answer.

A candidate may not proceed to the Objectively Structured Clinical Examination/Structured Oral Examination part of the Primary without passing the MCQ. An MCQ pass will be valid for a period of three years for a trainee working full time.

Although there is currently no limit on the number of attempts at this part of the examination, implicit in run through training is the need for trainees to achieve clinical competencies and examination milestones in a timely fashion.

It is generally acknowledged that an MCQ examination is a good test of core knowledge and there is no short cut to the acquisition of the considerable amount of information required to pass the Primary MCQ. Prospective candidates need to commit to an intensive programme of study of the syllabus supported by considerable practice of the technique of answering MCQs.

Dr Maclennan has produced a series of MCQs which cover in detail the Primary FRCA syllabus. The answer sections are clear and, where appropriate, supported by references to recent literature. Trainees commencing an anaesthesia training programme will find these MCQs useful to assess the depth of knowledge of the basic sciences which will be required of them, and those for whom the examination is imminent will find this series of books an invaluable means of self assessment and an indication of aspects of their knowledge and understanding which may need further work.

Dr D. Nolan, Regional Advisor for the North West

INTRODUCTION

Having taken both anaesthetic and medicine postgraduate examinations, I think that it is always difficult to know how best to start revising. It is important to avoid that unpleasant drowning sensation when you look at all the information that you have to absorb! I personally find that sitting and reading a textbook is time consuming, not particularly memorable and not especially useful for actually passing the exam. The best way to find out the gaps in your knowledge is to do as many practice MCQs as you can. This will stimulate you to read around the topics you are less familiar with, whilst improving your exam technique.

These books are different from others on the market as they are subject based. Many candidates feel that they have a particular area of weakness. These books will at worst highlight those weaknesses and at best, allow you to home in on specific topics, making them your areas of strength.

Each book contains 150 MCQs, covering pharmacology and clinical in book 1, physics, clinical measurement, equipment and statistics in book 2, physiology and anatomy in book 3. Within each book, the questions are mostly based in subject groups. This enables you to revise a particular topic or, you can always take a selection of questions from each book to make a practice exam paper.

The questions are based on the primary syllabus but will also be useful for candidates studying for the basic science part of the final examination.

Being pocket sized, there is now no excuse! Carry one in the pocket of your theatre blues and do a few questions before the patient arrives in the anaesthetic room or even over lunch!

The examination period is a stressful time, so make best use of *all* the time that you have.

Good luck!

Kirsty

Physics,

Clinical Measurement

and Equipment

MCQs

Indicate your answers with a tick or cross in the boxes provided.

2.1 Base SI units include:

☐ A Candela

☐ B Joule

☐ C Watt

☐ D Ohm

☐ E Amp

2.2 Derived SI units include:

☐ A Newton

☐ B Joule

☐ C Degree Celsius

☐ D Calorie

☐ E Atmosphere

2.1 Answers:

- A True
- B False
- C False
- D False
- E True

Base SI units include metre, kilogramme, second, ampere (amp), kelvin, candela and mole.

2.2 Answers:

- A True
- B True
- C True
- D False
- E False

From the seven base units numerous derived units may be obtained.

These include:

- for temperature – degrees Celsius
- for force – newton
- for pressure – pascal, bar
- for energy – joule or electronvolt
- for power – watt
- for frequency – hertz
- for volume – litre or cubic metre.

2.3   Regarding pressure, which of the following statements are true:

☐ A   Laplace's law for a sphere states $P = 2R \div T$, where P is the pressure gradient across the wall of a sphere, R is the radius and T is the tension

☐ B   Mean arterial pressure (MAP) could be as high as 27 kPa at the feet when standing

☐ C   MAP is estimated as: diastolic blood pressure + (systolic blood pressure – diastolic blood pressure) $\div$ 2

☐ D   Peripheral resistance = mean aortic blood pressure (if laminar flow is assumed) $\div$ cardiac output

☐ E   When measuring blood pressure, the width of the cuff should be 20% greater than the circumference of the arm

2.3 Answers:

- A False
- B True
- C False
- D True
- E False

Laplace's law for a spherical shape is: the pressure gradient across the wall of the sphere is $2T/R$.

Mean arterial pressure is: $(2 \times$ diastolic pressure$)$ + systolic pressure $\div 3$

or: diastolic pressure + (systolic – diastolic pressure) $\div 3$

When measuring blood pressure the cuff should be at the level of the heart.

The bladder should be over the brachial artery and the width of the cuff should be 20% greater than the diameter of the arm, not the circumference of the arm.

Reference: Yentis S.M. *Anaesthesia and Intensive Care A–Z*, 3rd edn. Butterworth–Heinemann, 2004.

2.4 **The following are true regarding non-invasive blood pressure monitoring:**

□ A The fifth phase of Korotkoff (ie final loss of sound during manual blood pressure monitoring) is widely accepted to indicate diastolic pressure

□ B When using a von Recklinghausen oscillotonometer the proximal cuff is wider than the distal, sensing cuff

□ C A standard adult cuff is designed to fit an arm circumference of 25–35 cm

□ D Automated oscillometric blood pressure machines usually have two cuffs, like the von Recklinghausen oscillotonometer

□ E When set to take regular readings, an automatic oscillometric blood pressure machine will inflate to 25 mmHg above the previous systolic measurement

2.4   Answers:

- A   True
- B   True
- C   True
- D   False
- E   True

Korotkoff (a Russian physician 1874–1920) originally described three phases.

These were subsequently increased to the five phases widely accepted today.

The Von Recklinghausen oscillotonometer comprises a proximal occluding cuff (5 cm wide) and a distal sensing cuff (10 cm wide).

The proximal occluding cuff is connected to a bellows, which is open to the atmosphere.

The distal sensing cuff is connected to a bellows closed from the atmosphere.

It is said to be reliable even at low pressures.

Most automated oscillometric machines have one cuff.

They initially inflate to a pressure of 160 mmHg and, when set to record at regular intervals, inflate to ~25 mmHg above the last systolic recording.

2.5   Regarding blood pressure monitoring:

☐ A The Penaz technique (finger blood pressure) relies on a photocell to measure infrared absorption of arterial blood

☐ B When using the Penaz technique a servo control is continuously inflating and deflating to keep the infrared absorption at a constant

☐ C Arterial catheters are continually flushed at a rate of 10 ml per hour

☐ D Systolic pressure is on average 5 mmHg lower with direct measurement compared with indirect measurement

☐ E The normal frequency range of arterial pressure wave is 0–20 Hz

2.5   Answers:

- A True
- B True
- C False
- D False
- E False

The Penaz technique is the continuous measure of finger blood pressure.

A finger cuff is initially calibrated to mean arterial blood pressure.

An infrared light-emitting diode (LED) and a photocell are then employed to calculate the amount of infrared (IR) absorbed by the arterial blood in the finger at mean arterial pressure.

As the volume of the blood in the finger increases during systole, the IR absorption increases and this information is fed to a servo control. The servo control inflates the cuff to return the absorption level back to that at initial calibration (mean arterial pressure). In this way, the pressure at the transducer gives a continuous trace of arterial pressure.

Arterial catheters are continuously flushed with heparinised or plain saline at a rate of 4 ml per hour.

Direct arterial measurement is normally approximately 5 mmHg higher when compared with indirect measurement.

A value of 0–40 Hz is the normal frequency range for the arterial pressure wave.

2.6 Resonance and damping (where D = the damping factor or the degree of damping):

☐ A Critical damping occurs when $D = 1$

☐ B Optimal damping is 0.6–0.7 of critical damping

☐ C A wide catheter raises the resonant frequency of the system

☐ D Another waveform with a frequency of less than 40 Hz will interfere with the blood pressure waveform

☐ E In a Wheatstone bridge circuit the null deflection of the galvanometer implies: $R1 \div R2 = R3 \div R4$ where $R3$ is a variable resistance and $R4$ is the resistance of a strain gauge transducer

2.6   Answers:

- A True
- B True
- C True
- D True
- E True

When a sudden change is imposed on a system, if no overshoot of the trace occurs then the system is said to be critically damped. Optimal damping is 0.6–0.7 of critical damping. In this case, if a sudden change is imposed on a system this degree of damping produces the fastest response without excessive oscillations.

An increase in the resonant frequency of the system occurs with short, wide, stiff catheters.

A frequency of less than 40 Hz will interfere with the blood pressure waveform because the frequency range for blood pressure is between 0 and 40 Hz.

Reference: Yentis SM. *Anaesthesia and Intensive Care A–Z*, 3rd edn. Butterworth–Heinemann, 2004.

2.7   Humidity:

☐ A In the upper trachea is 21 g/m^3

☐ B In the lower airways is 34 g/m^3

☐ C When measured with a hair hygrometer is accurate in detecting humidity between 30 and 90%

☐ D Is measured by blowing air through ether to determine the dew point in the Regnault's hygrometer

☐ E Can be assessed using UV light transmission

2.8   Regarding humidification devices:

☐ A Those devices that maintain relative humidity above 75% aid ciliary clearance in the trachea

☐ B Heat and moisture exchangers provide slightly less humidification compared with cold water baths

☐ C Under optimum conditions heat and moisture, exchangers can provide in excess of 25 g/m^3 humidity

☐ D Gas-driven or ultrasonic nebulisers work best when the size of water droplet is less than 1μm

☐ E Ultrasonic nebulizers routinely result in an absolute humidity of 150 g/m^3

2.7   Answers:

- A False
- B False
- C True
- D True
- E True

Humidity per 1 m^3 of air at 20°C is 17 g/m^3.

Humidity in the upper trachea at 34°C is 34 g/m^3.

Humidity in the lower trachea at 37°C is 44 g/m^3.

2.8   Answers:

- A True
- B False
- C True
- D False
- E False

Ciliary clearance starts to become abnormal if the relative humidity falls to less than 75%.

A list of humidification devices providing the lowest humidification first include:

- cold water bubble-through
- heat moisture exchangers
- heated water baths
- heated Bernoulli nebuliser and anvil
- ultrasonic nebulisers.

Regarding nebulised particle size:

- 20 μm particles are deposited in the tubing or upper respiratory tract.
- 5 μm particles fall out in the region of the trachea.
- Size 1 μm particles pass right through to the alveoli and are deposited there.

These are ideal for humidification.

Droplets of less than 1 μm are simply inhaled and then exhaled with minimal effect.

Ultrasonic nebulisers are adjustable but routinely provide approximately 80–90 g/m^3 absolute humidity.

2.9   Regarding oxygen measurement and pulse oximetry:

☐ A Central cyanosis becomes clinically detectable when the level of reduced haemoglobin reaches 0.5 g/dl

☐ B Beer's law states that each layer of equal thickness absorbs an equal fraction of radiation that passes through it

☐ C During oximetry, oxyhaemoglobin absorbs more red light at the wavelength 660 nm than deoxyhaemoglobin

☐ D Isosbestic points are solely dependent on haemoglobin concentration

☐ E Oxyhaemoglobin absorbs more infrared light at wavelength 940 nm than does deoxyhaemoglobin

2.10   Pulse oximetry:

☐ A Is made inaccurately high with HbF

☐ B Can give falsely low readings with methylene blue

☐ C Can give falsely low readings with carboxyhaemoglobin

☐ D Is accurate to ±2% (within a range of 70–100% saturation)

☐ E Is made inaccurate by hyperbilirubinaemia

2.9   Answers:

- A   False
- B   False
- C   False
- D   True
- E   True

Central cyanosis is clinically detectable when levels of reduced haemoglobin reach approximately 5 g/100 ml of blood.

Oxyhaemoglobin absorbs less light at wavelength 660 nm (red light) than does deoxyhaemoglobin.

At wavelength 940 nm (IR light) oxyhaemoglobin absorbs more light than does deoxyhaemoglobin.

Answer B is Lambert's law.

Beer's law states that the absorption of radiation by a given thickness of a solution of a given concentration is the same as that of twice the thickness of a solution of half the concentration.

2.10   Answers:

- A   False
- B   True
- C   False
- D   True
- E   False

Many factors make pulse oximetry inaccurate.

Inaccurately high readings are associated with carboxy-haemoglobin.

Inaccurately low readings are associated with methaemo-globinaemia, methylene blue and indocyanine green.

Bilirubin, sulph-haemoglobin and fetal haemoglobin do not alter the accuracy of pulse oximetry.

Reference: Measurement of pO_2, pCO_2, ph, pulse oximetry and capnography. *Anaesthesia and Intensive Care Medicine* 2002.

2.11   Regarding oxygen:

☐ A When assessing an arterial blood sample, the oxygen content is used as the main indicator of oxygenation

☐ B Van Slyke's apparatus is used to measure oxygen content in blood

☐ C Typical venous PO_2 is 5.33 kPa

☐ D The oxygen-combining power of fetal haemoglobin is greater than that of adult haemoglobin

☐ E Hüfner's constant is the volume of oxygen carried by 100 ml blood

2.11   Answers:

- A False
- B True
- C True
- D True
- E False

The assessment of oxygenation is based on the oxygen tension in kilopascals.

Van Slyke's apparatus and the Lex–O_2–Con apparatus both measure oxygen content.

The oxygen-combining power of fetal haemoglobin is greater than that of adult haemoglobin otherwise the fetus would be hypoxic.

Venous PO_2 of 5.33 kPa corresponds to 74% oxygen saturation on pulse oximetry.

Hüfner's constant is the volume of oxygen carried by 1 g haemoglobin and is commonly quoted as 1.39 or 1.34 ml.

The discrepancy is because some of the haemoglobin is in the form of methaemoglobin and cannot combine with oxygen.

2.12   The oxyhaemoglobin dissociation curve is shifted:

☐ A To the left with HbF (fetal haemoglobin)

☐ B To the left following acclimatisation

☐ C To the right during pregnancy

☐ D To the right by androgens

☐ E To the left by thyroxine

2.12   Answers:

- A False
- B False
- C True
- D True
- E False

50% value $= P_{50}$
75% value $=$ venous blood
97% value $=$ arterial blood

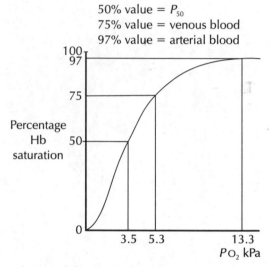

Figure: Oxyhaemoglobin dissociation curve

Factors shifting the curve to the left include a decrease in temperature, hydrogen ions, carbon dioxide and 2,3-DPG (2,3-diphosphoglycerate).

Increasing levels of carbon monoxide, fetal haemoglobin and methaemoglobin also shift the curve to the left.

Factors shifting the curve to the right include an increase in temperature, hydrogen ions, CO_2 and 2,3-DPG.

The following also shift the curve to the right, HbS, following acclimatisation, pregnancy, growth hormone, androgen and thyroxine.

2.13   Oxygen tension measurement:

☐ A Using Clark's electrode has a platinum cathode

☐ B Using Clark's electrode has potassium chloride or potassium hydroxide as the electrolyte solution

☐ C Using a fuel cell liberates electrons at the anode

☐ D Using a fuel cell may be made inaccurate when used in the presence of halothane

☐ E Using a fuel cell can be made inaccurate with concomitant use of nitrous oxide

2.14   Regarding paramagnetism:

☐ A If liquid oxygen is dropped into a magnetic field it would form a rotating ball in the centre of that field

☐ B The paramagnetism of oxygen is because the electrons in its outer shell are unpaired

☐ C Nitric oxide is paramagnetic

☐ D Nitrous oxide is diamagnetic

☐ E Paramagnetic analysers when used with null deflection analysers are, at best, accurate to $\pm 2\%$

2.13   Answers:

- A   True
- B   True
- C   True
- D   False
- E   True

Clark's electrode utilises a platinum cathode, a silver anode and either potassium hydroxide or potassium chloride as electrolyte solution.

It requires a battery to function (0.6 V).

This polarising voltage reduces the anaesthetic agent halothane and produces falsely high readings.

A fuel cell utilises lead as the anode and gold as the cathode with potassium hydroxide as the electrolyte solution.

Nitrous oxide reacts with lead in the presence of the electrolyte solution to produce nitrogen.

This alters the pressure inside the cell and may damage it.

Both the fuel cell and Clark's electrode liberate electrons at the anode.

Remember, anodes emit electrons and cathodes accept them.

2.14   Answers:

- A   True
- B   True
- C   True
- D   True
- E   False

Paramagnetic analysers used with null deflection analysers are accurate to $\pm 0.1\%$.

Diamagnetic substances are repelled by a magnetic field whereas paramagnetic substances are attracted to a magnetic field.

Unpaired electrons in the outer shell of oxygen render it paramagnetic.

2.15   Regarding electrical safety:

☐ A   It is recommended that the impedance of theatre shoes when new should be between 75 kΩ and 10 MΩ

☐ B   Theatre shoes should have a high enough impedance to prevent dissipation of electrostatic charges

☐ C   The patient is most at risk of ventricular fibrillation if an electrical impulse arrives at the heart during the R-wave of the ECG

☐ D   Any conducting part of a machine that can be touched by the user must be connected to earth in class I equipment

☐ E   Class II equipment has no need for parts accessible to the user to be connected to an earth wire

2.15   Answers:

- A True
- B False
- C False
- D True
- E True

Theatre shoes should have a high enough impedance to offer protection against electric shocks but a low enough impedance to allow dissipation of electrostatic charge. A patient is most at risk of an electric shock if it reaches the heart at the beginning of the T wave, ie during repolarisation.

Class I equipment has a non-communicating earth, neutral and live wire connected to a plug.

The additional safety feature is that the parts that can be touched by the user are connected to an earth wire.

If a fault occurs and the live wire comes into contact with these parts then a current flows from the live wire, eg through the metal case and then to an earth wire.

This current melts a protective fuse that disconnects the circuit.

Class II equipment (or double insulated) has no accessible parts that can conduct live current and so has no need for an earth wire.

Reference: *British Journal of Anaesthesia CEPD Reviews* 2003; 3(1): 10–14.

2.16 **With regard to electrical safety:**

☐ A Class III equipment can put the patient at risk of microshocks

☐ B Type CF equipment are suitable for use with electrical devices with direct cardiac connections

☐ C Type B equipment can be class I

☐ D Type BF equipment must have a maximum permitted leakage current not exceeding 200 µA

☐ E Type CF equipment must have a maximum permitted leakage current of less than 10 µA

Answers:

- A True
- B True
- C True
- D False
- E True

Although class III equipment uses safety extra-low voltage (SELV), which does not cause an electric shock, the patient is still at risk of microshock.

Because of this danger, latest standards relating to medical electrical equipment do not recognise class III.

Type B equipment may be of class I, II or III but the maximum leakage current must not exceed 100 μA.

It is therefore not suitable for direct connection to the heart.

Type C equipment has isolated circuits and offers the highest degree of protection. It is safe for connection to the heart.

There should be a maximum leakage current of less than 10 μA.

The letter F denotes that the circuit is floating, ie an earth-free or isolated circuit.

Reference: *British Journal of Anaesthesia CEPD Reviews* 2003; 3(1): 10–14.

2.17   Regarding electrical safety:

☐ A   Impedance of a capacitor is proportional to 1/frequency

☐ B   Impedance of an inductor is proportional to 1/frequency

☐ C   When connected to a current of 5 μA the patient may experience inability to let go of the faulty equipment

☐ D   The risk of asystole is great when connected to a current of 5 A

☐ E   100 μA is sufficient to cause ventricular fibrillation (VF) if delivered directly to the heart

2.17   Answers:

- A   True
- B   False
- C   False
- D   True
- E   True

Impedance is proportional to 1/frequency in a capacitor, whereas it is proportional to frequency in an inductor.

The series of symptoms for electrocution are as follows:

- 1 mA – tingling
- 5 mA – pain
- 15 mA – panic muscle contraction
- 50 mA – respiratory arrest
- 100 mA – VF
- >5 A – asystole.

However, in microshock, where current density is hugely important, the risk of VF can occur with current flows of 100 μA.

2.18 Regarding radiation and isotopes:

☐ A The atomic number is determined by the number of neutrons + protons

☐ B A positron is a positively charged β particle

☐ C A helium-4 nucleus is an example of an α particle

☐ D A γ ray has a high frequency and shortwave length

☐ E The SI unit of radioactivity is a curie

2.18   Answers:

- A False
- B True
- C True
- D True
- E False

An atomic number is determined by the number of protons, whereas the mass number is determined by the number of protons and neutrons contained within the nucleus.

A β particle (an electron) can be emitted during radioactive decay as can a positron (a positively charged beta particle).

An α particle can also be emitted, which is a combination of two protons + two neutrons (which is a helium-4 nucleus).

A γ ray (an electromagnetic wave) is usually emitted following radioactive decay.

A γ ray has high frequency and short wavelength.

The SI unit of radioactivity is the becquerel, ie a given quantity of radioactive substance has an activity of 1 becquerel (Bq) if one disintegration of a nucleus occurs on average every second.

A curie is the quantity of any radioactive substance undergoing 3.7×10^{10} disintegrations per second.

2.19 **Regarding lasers:**

☐ A The neodymium–YAG (yttrium–aluminium–garnet) laser is used for debulking tumours

☐ B When staff are utilising carbon dioxide lasers the risk of ocular damage is worse to the retina than to the cornea

☐ C The wavelength of the neodymium–YAG laser beam is greater than that of the argon laser beam

☐ D The carbon dioxide lasers need concurrent use of a helium laser to act as an aiming guide

☐ E The argon laser produces visible light

2.19   Answers:

- A   True
- B   False
- C   True
- D   True
- E   True

Laser (light amplification by stimulated emission of radiation) beams have five classic characteristics.

The light waves are:

- parallel
- monochromatic
- in phase
- non-divergent
- of high energy intensity produced with low power source.

Carbon dioxide lasers (wavelength 10 600 nm) emit infrared radiation and are absorbed within 200 μm of tissue, so the cornea is more at risk than the retina:

- They are used for precise surgery, cutting and coagulation.
- They require a helium laser to act as a guide in the visible spectrum.
- Argon or krypton lasers (400–700 nm) produce visible light.
- These lasers are used for photocoagulation especially in ophthalmology.
- Neodymium–YAG lasers, wavelength 1060 nm, are used for photocoagulation and debulking tumours.

2.20 Magnetic resonance (MR):

☐ A Magnets used in MR imaging (MRI) units have a magnetic flux density greater than 4 tesla

☐ B MRI detects the effects of magnetically induced changes in electrons of selected elements of the body

☐ C MR spectroscopy can be used to determine the relative abundance of certain substances locally in vivo

☐ D Aluminium cylinders are safe to use in an MR scanner

☐ E The only danger of ferromagnetic foreign bodies in a patient undergoing MRI is that the foreign body may move

2.21 In order for the following laws/hypothesis to be obeyed temperature must be at a constant:

☐ A Henry's law

☐ B Boyle's law

☐ C Charles' law

☐ D The third gas law

☐ E Avogadro's hypothesis

2.20 Answers:

- A False
- B False
- C True
- D True
- E False

Magnets used in an MRI unit have a magnetic flux density between 0.1 and 4 T.

The upper limit of magnetic flux density recommended for use is 4 T.

MRI detects effects of magnetically induced changes in nuclei, not electrons.

The danger of ferromagnetic foreign bodies includes not only risk of movement but also risk of burns secondary to the heating effect.

2.21 Answers:

- A True
- B True
- C False
- D False
- E True

Henry's law states that the amount of gas dissolved in a solvent is proportional to its partial pressure above the solvent at a constant temperature.

Boyle's law states that, at a constant temperature, the volume of a given mass of gas varies inversely with the absolute pressure.

Charles' law (or Gay Lussac's law) states that, at constant pressure, the volume of a given mass of gas varies directly with the absolute temperature.

The third gas law states that, at constant volume, the absolute pressure of a given mass of gas varies directly with the absolute temperature.

Avogadro's hypothesis states that equal volumes of gas at the same temperature and pressure contain equal numbers of molecules.

2.22 The following are true regarding gas laws and their applications:

☐ A An adiabatic change occurs when the state of the gas is altered without exchange of heat energy with its environment

☐ B Cryoprobes can create temperatures as low as −110°C

☐ C Nitrous oxide can be used in a cryoprobe

☐ D Dalton's law of partial pressures can be used to calculate alveolar carbon dioxide (once expired CO_2 percentage is known)

☐ E 38 g oxygen gas occupy 22.4 l at standard temperature and pressure

2.22   Answers:

- A True
- B False
- C True
- D True
- E False

Cryoprobes utilise the physics of adiabatic change.

Nitrous oxide and carbon dioxide can be used in cryoprobes and the lowest temperature attainable is −70°C.

Dalton's law of partial pressures states that the pressure exerted by each gas in a mixture of gases is the same as that which it would exert if it alone occupied the container.

If the percentage of expired carbon dioxide is known, once saturated vapour pressure of water is deducted, the partial pressure of alveolar carbon dioxide can then be calculated from atmospheric pressure.

Option E requires knowledge of Avogadro's number, ie that 1 mole of gas occupies 22.4 l at standard temperature and pressure.

Oxygen exists as O_2; 1 mole has an atomic mass of 16×2, which equals 32 g not 38 g.

2.23   Regarding gas laws:

☐   A   The critical temperature is the temperature above which a substance exists only as a gas

☐   B   The critical temperature of CO_2 is 36.5°C

☐   C   The critical pressure of oxygen is 60 bars

☐   D   The critical pressure of carbon dioxide is 70 bars

☐   E   The critical pressure of nitrous oxide is 75 bars

2.24   Regarding temperatures:

☐   A   The triple point of water is 273.15 K (kelvin)

☐   B   At absolute zero an ideal gas is predicted to occupy zero volume

☐   C   Mercury thermometers equilibrate in 1 minute

☐   D   Mercury freezes at −20°C

☐   E   Alcohol freezes at −100°C

2.23 **Answers:**

- A True
- B False
- C False
- D False
- E False

The critical temperature is the temperature above which a substance cannot be liquefied by pressure alone.

The critical pressure is the pressure required to liquefy a vapour at its critical temperature.

Gas	Critical temperature (°C)	Critical pressure (bars)
Oxygen	−118	50
Nitrous oxide	36.5	72
Carbon dioxide	31	73

2.24 **Answers:**

- A False
- B True
- C False
- D False
- E False

Temperature in K = temperature in °C + 273.15.

Triple point of water is 0.01°C, ie 273.16 K.

Mercury thermometers take 2–3 minutes to equilibrate, which is one of their drawbacks.

Their more serious drawback is the fact that mercury is poisonous.

Mercury freezes at −39°C and boils at over 250°C.

Alcohol freezes at −117°C and boils at 78.5°C.

2.25   Regarding temperature measurement:

☐ A Use of a resistance thermometer relies on the fact that the resistance of a platinum wire increases exponentially with an increase in temperature

☐ B Use of a thermistor, containing a metal oxide semi-conducting bead, is easily calibrated

☐ C Use of a thermocouple relies on the Seebeck effect

☐ D Use of large thermocouples gives a faster response time

☐ E Use of a thermocouple produces voltage at both reference and measuring junctions

2.25   Answers:

- A False
- B False
- C True
- D False
- E True

A platinum wire is an example of a resistance thermometer.

Its resistance increases linearly with increasing temperature.

The metal oxide bead is an example of a thermistor.

Its resistance falls exponentially with increase in temperature.

They are difficult to calibrate.

The response time of a thermocouple is very fast, particularly if the measuring probe is small ranging from 0.1 to 15 seconds.

Thermocouples operate on the principle of the Seebeck effect, whereby a small voltage is produced at the junction of two dissimilar metals, depending on the temperature at the junction.

There are two junctions within the circuit, one acting as a reference (kept at a constant temperature) and the other measuring, for example, patient temperature.

As the temperature at the measuring junction increases, the voltage flow increases.

2.26   Body temperature:

☐   A   Is commonly measured by UV thermometry when using a tympanic temperature-measuring device

☐   B   When measured rectally is normally slightly lower than core

☐   C   Average patient temperature equals one-third core temperature plus two-thirds average skin temperature

☐   D   Is increased by shivering, which increases the energy expenditure of an average sized male to approximately 100 W, ie 100 J/s

☐   E   One-quarter of heat loss secondary to respiration is due to warming of the air

2.26   Answers:

- A   False
- B   False
- C   False
- D   False
- E   True

Infrared thermometry is used to calculate tympanic temperatures, which relate accurately to hypothalamic temperature.

Rectal temperature is normally 0.5–1°C higher than core temperature.

This is secondary to bacterial fermentation in the stool.

Average patient temperature equals one-third average skin temperature plus two-thirds core temperature.

Shivering increases the heat production by up to fourfold from the usual 80 W to approximately 320 W.

Only 25% of respiratory heat loss is secondary to warming of the air; the rest is spent on humidification of the air.

2.27   Regarding specific heat capacity:

☐ A The definition for heat capacity is the amount of heat required to raise the temperature of 1 kg of a substance by 1 K

☐ B The mean value for the tissue specific heat capacity of a person is 3.5 kJ/kg per °C

☐ C 4.18 J are required to raise the temperature of 1 kg of water by 1°C

☐ D Gases have very low specific heat capacity

☐ E Radiation is proportional to the fourth power of the absolute temperature

2.28   Regarding heat/temperature:

☐ A The latent heat of vaporisation of water decreases linearly with an increase in temperature

☐ B The latent heat of vaporisation of nitrous oxide is zero at 36.5°C

☐ C As nitrous oxide flows from a cylinder, the vapour pressure within the cylinder falls because of cooling

☐ D Increasing temperature increases the viscosity of gases

☐ E Increasing temperature increases the viscosity of liquids

2.27   Answers:
- A False
- B True
- C False
- D True
- E True

Specific heat capacity is defined as the amount of heat required to raise the temperature of 1 kg of a substance by 1 K, whereas heat capacity relates to the temperature required to raise the temperature of a given object (not necessarily 1 kg weight).

The low specific heat capacity of gases can be attributed to their low density.

The value 4.18 kJ/kg per °C is the specific heat capacity of water.

Radiation (*R*) is proportional to the fourth power of the absolute temperature (AT).

(You either do or do not know this!)

2.28   Answers:
- A False
- B True
- C True
- D True
- E False

The latent heat of vaporisation of water does not decrease linearly with increase in temperature.

The graph is curved.

The latent heat of vaporisation of a substance is zero at its critical temperature.

Nitrous oxide takes heat energy from the liquid nitrous oxide and the cylinder to become a vapour.

In doing so, the pressure within the cylinder falls and the vapour pressure decreases because of this cooling.

Viscosity of a gas increases with increasing energy as more movement occurs.

With liquids, increasing energy reduces van der Waals' forces and therefore decreases viscosity.

2.29   Regarding hydrogen ions and their measurement:

☐   A   A pH of 7.6 has 76 nmol/l H^+

☐   B   Approximately 13 000 mmol hydrogen ions are produced by the body per day

☐   C   The hydrogen ion electrode is accurate without a thermal control system

☐   D   The reference electrode of a hydrogen ion electrode is made of the same material as the anode of Clark's electrode

☐   E   The hydrogen ion electrode is calibrated with two buffer solutions containing fixed concentrations of two phosphate buffers

2.30   When measuring carbon dioxide with the Severinghaus electrode:

☐   A   It measures carbon dioxide directly

☐   B   pH changes linearly with log CO_2

☐   C   It is accurate to 1 mmHg, which is written $mmHgCO_2$

☐   D   The response time is faster than that of the hydrogen electrode

☐   E   The electrode has a plastic membrane impermeable to CO_2, which separates the liquid to be tested from the bicarbonate solution

2.29 **Answers:**
- A False
- B True
- C False
- D True
- E True

A pH of 7.6 is 60 nmol/l hydrogen ions, whereas a pH of 7.4 is 40 nmol/l hydrogen ions.

Acids and bases dissociate at increased speed at high temperatures, so the measurement of hydrogen ions must be at 37°C and a correction factor must be applied if the patient is not normothermic.

Both Clark's electrode and the reference electrode of the hydrogen electrode are made of Ag/AgCl.

The fuel cell anode is made of lead.

2.30 **Answers:**
- A False
- B True
- C True
- D False
- E False

The Severinghaus electrode measures hydrogen ion change, not CO_2 directly.

The electrode works on the basis that $CO_2 + H_2O$ combine to give H_2CO_3 which gives $H^+ + HCO_3^-$.

The electrode has a number of components.

Initially the liquid to be tested is separated from the electrode by a plastic membrane permeable to CO_2.

CO_2 diffuses across this membrane and reacts with the water of the bicarbonate solution.

H^+ and HCO_3^- ions are produced.

H^+ then diffuses through the H^+-sensitive glass, whereupon it is measured by the glass electrode.

The hydrogen electrode has a faster response time, as it is not reliant upon CO_2 diffusion and reaction before measurement.

2.31   Regarding infrared carbon dioxide measurement:

☐ A Carbon dioxide maximally absorbs infrared wavelength
4.28 μm

☐ B Physiological or 0.9% saline absorbs infrared radiation

☐ C Sapphire blocks infrared radiation

☐ D Collision broadening is an effect whereby energy from infrared
absorption can be transmitted to another dissimilar molecule

☐ E Temperature can affect the infrared absorption of molecules

2.32   Regarding carbon dioxide analysers:

☐ A Side-stream analysers siphon off gas at a rate of 50 ml/min

☐ B The side-stream analyser sample line must be less than
2 metres in length

☐ C The rise time is the time taken for the reading in the analyser to
change from 10% to 90% of the final value

☐ D Too high a flow of gas in the sampling line of the side-stream
analyser could cause a significant pressure drop across the
sampling line, leading to inaccuracies

☐ E Metacresol purple dye changes from yellow to purple when
exposed to carbon dioxide

2.31 Answers:
- A True
- B False
- C False
- D True
- E False

Carbon dioxide maximally absorbs infrared radiation at wavelength 4.28 μm.

Nitrous oxide absorbs infrared radiation between 4.4 and 4.5 μm.

Glass absorbs infrared radiation whereas 0.9% saline and sapphire do not.

Collision broadening can be experienced with carbon dioxide and nitrous oxide.

As carbon dioxide molecules absorb infrared radiation it gains energy.

This energy can be transferred to nitrous oxide molecules, which leave the carbon dioxide free to absorb more infrared radiation.

This makes the monitored concentration of carbon dioxide inaccurately high.

2.32 Answers:
- A False
- B True
- C True
- D True
- E False

Side-stream analysers siphon gas off at a rate of approximately 150 ml/min.

Flow less than this leads to a slow transit time, which will have an effect on rise time.

High flow leads to incorrect results secondary to decreased pressure in the sample line (the output of the analyser depends on pressure).

Metacresol purple changes from purple to yellow with carbon dioxide and can be used in emergencies when capnography is not available.

2.33   Regarding diffusion:

☐   A   Fick's law of diffusion states that the rate of diffusion of a substance is proportional to the thickness of the membrane

☐   B   The diffusion of a gas across a membrane into a liquid is proportional to its solubility in that liquid

☐   C   Oxygen is more soluble in tissues than carbon dioxide

☐   D   The equilibration of oxygen between alveolar to capillaries takes 0.75 s

☐   E   The diffusion of volatile gases resembles carbon dioxide diffusion in relation to speed

2.34   Diffusion capacity:

☐   A   Is measured using carbon monoxide

☐   B   Is dependent on pulmonary blood flow

☐   C   Is halved postpneumonectomy

☐   D   Can be a measure of disease severity in sarcoidosis

☐   E   Is increased in cardiac failure

2.33   Answers:

- A   False
- B   True
- C   False
- D   False
- E   True

Fick's law of diffusion states that the rate of diffusion of a substance across a unit area is proportional to the concentration gradient.

Oxygen is less soluble in tissues than carbon dioxide.

Blood in pulmonary capillaries passes through an alveolus in approximately 0.75 s.

Oxygen equilibrates in approximately 0.3–0.4 s whereas CO_2 equilibrates within approximately 0.1 s.

CO_2 and volatile agents have very similar solubilities.

2.34   Answers:

- A   True
- B   False
- C   True
- D   True
- E   False

Diffusion capacity is measured using carbon monoxide.

Carbon monoxide is hugely soluble in blood, so the carbon monoxide tension in the pulmonary capillaries is assumed to be zero.

The rate of diffusion of carbon monoxide is therefore not dependent on pulmonary blood flow.

The rate is dependent on the speed of diffusion across the membrane.

Pneumonectomy halves the diffusion capacity.

Anything that thickens the membrane would decrease the diffusion capacity including oedema (heart failure).

2.35   Diffusion:
- ☐ A When using nitrous oxide in an intubated patient, care should be taken to monitor endotracheal (ET) tube cuff pressure
- ☐ B Graham's law states that the rate of diffusion of a gas is inversely proportional to its molecular weight
- ☐ C The diffusion of a gas across a membrane is proportional to the tension gradient
- ☐ D Nitrous oxide is more soluble in blood with increasing pressures
- ☐ E Henry's law is temperature dependent

2.36   Regarding osmosis and osmolality:
- ☐ A A pure semipermeable membrane is freely permeable to solvents
- ☐ B One mole of solute dissolved in 22.4 l of solvent exerts an osmotic pressure of 101.325 kPa
- ☐ C One mole of large solute molecules exerts greater osmotic pressure compared with one mole of small solute molecules across a semipermeable membrane
- ☐ D Osmolality is measured in milliosmoles per kilogram of water or other solvent
- ☐ E Osmolarity is measured in milliosmoles per kilogram of water

2.35   Answers:

- A   True
- B   False
- C   True
- D   True
- E   True

Nitrous oxide can easily diffuse into the air inside an ET tube cuff; therefore, during long cases when using nitrous oxide, cuff pressure should be monitored.

Graham's law states that the rate of diffusion of a gas is inversely proportional to the square root of its molecular mass.

Henry's law states that at a particular temperature the amount of a given gas dissolved in a given liquid is directly proportional to the partial pressure of the gas in equilibrium with the liquid.

2.36   Answers:

- A   True
- B   True
- C   False
- D   True
- E   False

A pure semipermeable membrane is freely permeable to solvent but is impermeable to solute.

Option B is correct. Equally, 1 mole of perfect gas in a volume of 22.4 l exerts a pressure of 1 atmosphere.

Provided that the membrane is impermeable to the solute the size of the molecules is irrelevant to the osmotic pressure exerted.

Osmolality is measured in mosmol/kg of water or other solvent whereas osmolarity is measured in mosmol/l of solution.

In research, osmolality is used as it avoids inaccuracies secondary to the temperature effect on the volume of solution.

2.37   Hartmann's solution contains:

☐ A Potassium 3.5 mmol/l

☐ B Calcium 5 mmol/l

☐ C Magnesium 2 mmol/l

☐ D Lactate 27 mmol/l

☐ E Osmolarity 270 mosmol/l

2.38   Regarding oncotic pressure and osmolarities:

☐ A Plasma proteins exert approximately 6% of the osmolarity of plasma

☐ B Red cell fragility test identifies abnormal red blood cells as they burst at lower osmolarities

☐ C Capillary oncotic pressure is approximately 6 kPa at the arterial end

☐ D A fall in plasma oncotic pressure by 40% leads to oedema

☐ E Oncotic pressure is measured with a tonconometer

2.37   Answers:

- A False
- B False
- C False
- D False
- E False

1 litre of Hartmann's solution contains:

- sodium 131 mmol
- chloride 111 mmol
- lactate 29 mmol
- potassium 5 mmol
- calcium 2 mmol.

The sum of all these components is the osmolarity, which is 278 mosmol/l.

2.38   Answers:

- A False
- B True
- C False
- D True
- E False

Plasma proteins exert very little effect on the osmolarity of plasma exerting only 1 mosmol/l.

They exert an oncotic pressure of approximately 3.5 kPa, predominantly secondary to albumin.

A fall in oncotic pressure to approximately 2 kPa (ie a 40% drop) is enough to cause oedema.

Oncotic pressure is measured using an oncometer.

Red cell fragility test is used to detect abnormal red cells.

At low osmolarities water dissolves into the red blood cell.

At a critical hydrostatic pressure within the red blood cell it will burst.

Abnormal blood cells burst at lower hydrostatic pressures.

2.39   Regarding osmolality measurement:

☐   A   An osmometer measures osmolality

☐   B   One mole of substance added to one kilogram of water increases the freezing point by 1.86°C

☐   C   Increasing solute load causes depression of the freezing point

☐   D   Raoult's law states that depression of the vapour pressure of a solvent is proportional to the molar concentration of the solute

☐   E   Osmometers utilising Raoult's law are advantageous as smaller samples can be tested

2.40   The saturated vapour pressure:

☐   A   Is the partial pressure of vapour above a liquid in a closed container at equilibrium

☐   B   Of an anaesthetic agent is an indicator of its volatility

☐   C   Of diethyl ether is lower than that of halothane

☐   D   Is always constant for a substance

☐   E   At boiling point is greater than atmospheric pressure

2.39   Answers:

- A   False
- B   False
- C   True
- D   True
- E   True

Osmometers calculate osmolality, based on the principle that depression of the freezing point of a solution is directly proportional to its osmolality.

One mole of a substance added to one kilogram of water depresses freezing point by 1.86°C.

Osmometers utilising Raoult's principle rather than depression of the freezing point are advantageous as they only require small samples to be tested and so can be used to test, for example, sweat.

Raoult's law states that the depression or lowering of vapour pressure of a solvent is proportional to the molar concentration of the solute.

2.40   Answers:

- A   True
- B   True
- C   False
- D   False
- E   False

The saturated vapour pressure of diethyl ether is 59 kPa compared with halothane at 32 kPa. (Note: do not confuse with ethyl chloride.)

Saturated vapour pressure is not always constant but is dependent upon temperature.

At boiling point, the saturated vapour pressure is equal to atmospheric pressure.

Saturated vapour pressure increases with temperature, so saturated vapour pressures of volatile agents are quoted at standard temperature, usually 20°C.

2.41   Regarding solubilities:

☐ A Henry's law states that the amount of gas dissolved in a given liquid is directly proportional to the partial pressure of gas in equilibrium with a liquid at a given temperature

☐ B Gases are more soluble in warm liquids

☐ C Nitrous oxide is more soluble in water than nitrogen

☐ D The Ostwald solubility coefficient is measured at standard temperature and pressure

☐ E The Bunsen solubility coefficient is most commonly used in anaesthetic practice

2.41   Answers:

- A True
- B False
- C True
- D False
- E False

Clearly, gases are less soluble in warm liquids as is seen when water boils.

Nitrous oxide is more soluble than nitrogen in water and in blood.

The Ostwald solubility coefficient is the volume of gas that dissolves in one unit volume of the liquid at the temperature and pressure concerned, whereas the Bunsen solubility coefficient is measured at standard temperature and pressure.

The Ostwald solubility coefficient is commonly used in anaesthetic practice, as the patients are not at 'standard temperature'.

2.42   Regarding solubility:

☐ A Partition coefficients are defined as a ratio

☐ B Partition coefficients are different to Ostwald solubility
      coefficients as they can be applied to two liquids

☐ C Nitrous oxide is more soluble in oil than blood

☐ D A volatile anaesthetic agent with a high Ostwald solubility
      coefficient will have a rapid speed of onset

☐ E The Ostwald solubility coefficient for nitrous oxide in 1 litre of
      blood is 0.47 at 37°C and atmospheric pressure

2.42   Answers:

- A   True
- B   True
- C   True
- D   False
- E   True

Partition coefficient is defined as the ratio of the amount of substance present in one phase compared with another, the two phases being of equal volume and in equilibrium. At 37°C, 1.4 l nitrous oxide will dissolve in 1 l oil compared with 0.47 l nitrous oxide that will dissolve in 1 l blood.

A high Ostwald solubility coefficient indicates that the volatile agent is very soluble in blood.

The anaesthetic agent is easily carried away from the lungs, so the alveolar concentration builds up very slowly and there is slow onset of anaesthesia. Some examples of Ostwald solubility coefficients are as follows:

- xenon 0.14
- nitrous oxide 0.47
- desflurane 0.45
- sevoflurane 0.69
- isoflurane 1.4
- enfrane 1.8
- halothane 2.4.

That is, desflurane with a low Ostwald solubility coefficient will have a faster onset of action than halothane with a high Ostwald solubility coefficient.

Reference: Peck TE, Williams M. *Pharmacology for Anaesthesia and Intensive Care*. Greenwich Medical Media Ltd., 2003.

2.43 Regarding minimum alveolar concentration (MAC) and anaesthetic agents:

☐ A MAC is the measure of solubility of an anaesthetic agent in blood

☐ B A substance with a high MAC is highly potent

☐ C The MAC value for nitrous oxide is derived from animal studies

☐ D Malignant hyperpyrexia maybe triggered by absorbed anaesthetic vapour in a circuit

☐ E A low MAC indicates fast speed of onset of an anaesthetic agent

2.43   Answers:

- A False
- B False
- C False
- D True
- E False

MAC represents the solubility of an agent in oil, the MAC 50 being the level above which 50% of patients cease to move in response to a standard surgical stimulus.

MAC is inversely related to anaesthetic potency.

The MAC value for nitrous oxide (over 100%) is theoretical, based on the partial pressure of nitrous oxide when used in a pressure chamber.

Speed of onset is determined by the blood : gas partition coefficient.

An agent with a low blood : gas partition coefficient has a more rapid onset and offset.

2.44   Chromatography:

☐ A Can be used to measure the concentrations of anaesthetic
        agents in a mixture

☐ B Is commonly used in clinical anaesthetic practice

☐ C Can make use of calcium carbonate (among other compounds)
        to form a mobile phase

☐ D Requires large particles to form the stationary phase in gas
        chromatography

☐ E Does not require strict temperature control

2.44   Answers:

- A True
- B False
- C False
- D False
- E False

Chromatography is predominantly used in laboratories and is not routinely used in theatre or clinical areas.

It enables gases and liquids to be both identified and measured in a mixture.

It consists of two fundamental phases – the stationary phase is composed of solid compounds, eg carbon carbonate in liquid chromatography and silica aluminium in gas chromatography.

The mobile phase is composed of a carrier gas, eg helium, argon or nitrogen.

Very small particles are needed to form the stationary phase in gas chromatography to enable differentiation of the gases.

Temperature control is extremely important, as solubility is temperature dependent.

The column is maintained at specific temperatures in, for example, ovens.

2.45   Regarding gas chromatography:
- ☐ A Separation of gases occurs depending on their densities
- ☐ B A katharometer is an example of a suitable detector for analysis of oxygen
- ☐ C Blood samples can be analysed by gas chromatography
- ☐ D It enables continuous analysis
- ☐ E It allows the identification of very low concentrations of drugs

2.46   Regarding gas chromatography detectors:
- ☐ A A flame ionisation detector is used to detect organic vapours
- ☐ B A flame ionisation detector utilises a nitrogen flame burning in air
- ☐ C A flame ionisation detector is able to identify unknown substances
- ☐ D A katharometer is useful for detecting inorganic vapours
- ☐ E Electron capture detectors are useful for detecting halogenated compounds

2.45   Answers:

- A   False
- B   True
- C   True
- D   False
- E   True

The separation of gases is dependent upon their different solubility in the two phases (ie stationary and mobile), which is why temperature control is so important.

Blood samples can be analysed but first must be vaporised.

Katharometers are discussed below.

Continuous chromatographic analysis is impossible.

2.46   Answers:

- A   True
- B   False
- C   False
- D   True
- E   True

There are three main detectors – flame ionisation detectors, katharometers and electron capture detectors.

The principle of the flame ionisation detector is that a flame of hydrogen gas burning in air has a potential difference applied across it.

Organic vapour applied to the gas stream causes a change in current flow proportional to the amount of substance present.

Katharometers are thermal conductivity detectors (gas changes the electrical resistance of a heated wire) and are useful in inorganic gas detection, eg nitrous oxide and oxygen.

Electron capture detectors again utilise a polarised voltage, which is applied across an ionisation chamber.

Halogenated compounds capture these electrons so reducing current flow.

2.47   Regarding mass spectrometry:

☐ A Substances are analysed according to their molecular mass

☐ B Electrons arising from an anode charge the particles in the ionisation chamber

☐ C It cannot be used for online gas analysis during anaesthesia

☐ D Knowledge of cracking pattern can aid identification

☐ E It requires relatively large sample sizes for identification

2.47   Answers:

- A True
- B False
- C False
- D True
- E False

The process of mass spectrometry is as follows:

1. Sample is actively drawn into a sample chamber.
2. Sample is bombarded with electrons in an ionisation chamber emitted from a hot cathode.
3. Charged particles are accelerated out of a chamber by means of plates generating an electric field.
4. The charged particles pass through a strong magnetic field.
5. Different deflection of particles according to their mass and momentum allows identification.

Compounds with identical masses, eg nitrous oxide and carbon dioxide, can be identified by quadruple mass spectrometry. With this method, the accelerated beam is passed longitudinally among four rods of viable potential. All particles are removed from the beam of accelerated ions, which are not of a specific mass. This enables identification of breakdown products, ie cracking pattern. A great advantage of mass spectrometry is the need for only very small samples. Response time can be as quick as 100 ms.

2.48 Regarding vapour analysis:

☐ A Piezo-electric effect can be used to measure vapour concentration

☐ B Raman spectrometry can be used to analyse single atoms

☐ C Raman spectrometry can be used to perform multiple simultaneous gas analysis

☐ D Raman spectrometry is as accurate as mass spectrometry

☐ E Hook and Tucker analysis is used to detect isoflurane

2.48   Answers:

- A   True
- B   False
- C   True
- D   True
- E   False

Piezo-electric effect is a phenomenon whereby a quartz crystal contracts when exposed to an electric potential. These crystals are coated in oil and are then set to oscillate at their resonant frequency.

Anaesthetic vapour dissolves in the oil and alters the frequency of oscillations.

Raman spectrometry relies on the molecules' effect on the wavelength of light.

A specific wavelength of light radiation causes a specific energy transfer to the molecule.

This transfer of energy causes a decrease in the radiation wavelength, which is specific to that gas and concentration.

The Raman effect can therefore be used to measure partial pressures of a range of gases. A powerful light source must be used, eg argon laser.

To produce a signal that is able to be detected signal atoms cannot be detected by this method.

Hook and Tucker analysis depends on the ability of halothane to absorb UV light.

2.49   Regarding combustions:

☐ A A stoichiometric concentration by definition
         vapour or oxidising agent once a combustic
         complete

☐ B Stoichiometric concentrations differ in oxygen and air

☐ C An explosion is more violent with pure oxygen present than
         with oxygen and nitrous oxide

☐ D Liquid spirit burns with a pale blue flame

☐ E Category Anaesthetic-Proof (AP) equipment can be used in a
         zone that contains a flammable anaesthetic mixture with
         oxygen or nitrous oxide

2.50   Regarding force:

☐ A The (derived) SI unit of force is the kilogram weight

☐ B One newton equals one kilogram per metre

☐ C The force of gravity on a 1 kg object will cause an acceleration
         of 9.81 m/s^2

☐ D The (derived) SI unit of pressure (pascal) is defined as the
         pressure of 1 N activity over an area of 1 m^2

☐ E It is the area multiplied by the pressure

Answers:

- A True
- B True
- C False
- D True
- E False

Combustion of nitrous oxide releases energy and oxygen ($2N_2O$ goes to $2N_2 + O_2$ + energy), so causing a more violent explosion than oxygen alone.

Option E refers to APG-labelled equipment.

AP equipment can be used only in a zone that contains a flammable anaesthetic mixture with air, ie not oxygen or nitrous oxide.

Anaesthetic Proof Category G (APG) equipment does not present a risk of ignition of a flammable anaesthetic mixture with oxygen or nitrous oxide; it can be used within 5 cm of gas escaping from a breathing system.

If equipment is not labelled it should be assumed unsafe to use around flammable gas mixtures.

2.50 Answers:

- A False
- B False
- C True
- D True
- E True

The derived SI unit of force is the newton (N), which will give a mass of one kilogram an acceleration of one metre per second per second, ie 1 N = 1 kg/m per s^2.

The SI unit of pressure is the pascal, which is the pressure of 1 N/m^2.

Pressure equals force (measured in newtons) divided by area (in metres squared), ie $P = F \div A$.

2.51   **The following are true of the physics of valves:**

☐ A Pressure-relieving valves open when the exerted pr.. sufficient to overcome the force that the spring exerts ov.. disc

☐ B Pressure-regulating (reducing) valves control the supply of oxygen from the cylinders

☐ C In pressure-regulating (reducing) valves the force of the spring equals the force acting on the conical valve + the force acting on a diaphragm

☐ D Pressure-regulating (reducing) valves have many similar features to the oxygen-failure warning devices

☐ E The second stage of the entonox valve is identical to a pressure-reducing valve

2.52   **One atmosphere is equal to:**

☐ A 1000 kPa

☐ B 102 cmH$_2$O

☐ C 7.6 mmHg

☐ D 1 bar

☐ E 10^5 N/m^2

.51   Answers:

- A   True
- B   True
- C   True
- D   True
- E   False

Pressure-relieving valves allow excess pressure to be released from a system.

Once a pressure reaches a set limit, the force of the spring acting on a diaphragm is overcome and gas is allowed to escape until the preset pressure is reached.

Pressure-reducing valves tend to open secondary to a fall in pressure in the system.

With a fall in pressure, the force of a spring acting on a diaphragm dislodges an occlusive stopper.

This allows gas to enter into the area under the diaphragm, until the pressure under the diaphragm is sufficient to overcome the force of the spring and raise the stopper back to its original position.

The first stage of an entonox valve is a pressure-reducing valve.

2.52   Answers:

- A   False
- B   False
- C   False
- D   True
- E   True

One atmosphere equals:

- 101.325 kPa
- 1020 cmH$_2$O
- 750 mmHg
- 1 bar.

2.53   Regarding pressure measurement:

☐   A   The absolute pressure of an empty oxygen cylinder is 0 bar

☐   B   The pressure in water at 10.2 cm depth will always be
        10.2 g/cm^2

☐   C   Mercury barometers measure absolute pressure

☐   D   Low-density liquids increase inaccuracy in manometers

☐   E   10.2 cmH$_2$O pressure is 1 bar

2.54   Regarding laminar flow:

☐   A   Flow is mass or volume multiplied by time

☐   B   It has a central flow four times as fast as mean flow

☐   C   No flow occurs as fluid approaches the walls of the vessel

☐   D   A linear relationship exists between pressure and flow

☐   E   Halving the tube diameter decreases flow by eightfold

2.53   Answers:

- A   False
- B   True
- C   True
- D   False
- E   False

Option A refers to relative or gauge pressure.

The absolute pressure of an empty cylinder of oxygen is atmospheric pressure, ie 1 bar at sea level.

Otherwise the cylinder would collapse.

Mercury barometers are sealed and measure absolute pressure.

Low-density liquids increase the accuracy of manometers.

10.2 cmH_2O pressure is one-hundredth of a bar.

2.54   Answers:

- A   False
- B   False
- C   True
- D   True
- E   False

Flow is quantity of a fluid passing a certain point per unit time, ie mass or volume ÷ time.

Central flow is twice that of mean flow in laminar flow.

Halving the diameter decreases the flow to one-sixteenth of its original value.

2.55 Relating to laminar flow:

☐ A Flow is directly proportional to viscosity

☐ B Flow is directly proportional to density

☐ C Flow is indirectly proportional to the distance that the fluid travels

☐ D Flow is doubled if the diameter is doubled

☐ E It has eddies

2.56 Regarding turbulent flow in tubes that are rough on the inside:

☐ A Flow is directly proportional to the pressure

☐ B To double the flow pressure must be trebled

☐ C Flow is directly proportional to 1 divided by the length of the tube

☐ D Flow is indirectly proportional to 1 divided by the square root of the density of the fluid

☐ E The graph plotted for pressure and flow would be a parabola

2.55 Answers:

- A False
- B False
- C True
- D False
- E False

Remember laminar flow obeys the Hagen–Poiseuille equation of flow:

$P\pi d^4 \div 128\eta l$

where P = pressure difference across the tube, d = diameter of tube, η = viscosity and l = length of tube.

Flow is directly proportional to the pressure difference across the tube and the diameter to the power of 4.

Flow is indirectly proportional to the viscosity and the length of the tube.

Density becomes important in turbulent flow.

Laminar flow has neither eddies nor turbulence.

2.56 Answers:

- A False
- B False
- C False
- D False
- E True

During turbulent flow, flow is approximately proportional to the square root of the pressure.

To double flow pressure must be increased by a factor of 4.

Flow is directly proportional to 1 divided by the square root of the length of the tube and 1 divided by the square root of the density of the fluid.

The relationship between pressure and flow is non-linear and when plotted forms a parabola obeying formula:

$y = a + bx + cx^2$.

Where y and x are the variables pressure and flow, and a, b and c are the parameters.

2.57   Reynolds' number:

☐ A Is dimensionless

☐ B Is greater with a more viscous fluid

☐ C Above 2000 is more likely to result in turbulent flow

☐ D Is altered when breathing helium compared with air because of a reduction in viscosity

☐ E Can be calculated only if the length of the tube is known

2.57   Answers:

- A True
- B False
- C True
- D False
- E False

Reynolds' number is a dimensionless number used to calculate when the flow of a fluid becomes turbulent.

Reynolds' number = density × velocity × diameter of tube ÷ viscosity:

$\rho v d \div \eta$

If the result exceeds 2000 turbulent flow is more likely.

The point at which laminar flow becomes turbulent occurs at a critical velocity.

This critical velocity is specific for that fluid in that tube.

The beneficial effect of helium on an obstructed airway is secondary to its low density not viscosity.

Its low density reduces Reynolds' number and so reduces turbulence.

2.58   Regarding fluid flow:

☐   A   Breathing air decreases the risk of turbulent airway flow as opposed to breathing an oxygen: nitrous oxide mix

☐   B   The predominant effect of warming and humidifying inspired gases is to increase density and therefore turbulence

☐   C   Turbulent flow predominates in the lower respiratory tract

☐   D   Tension is measured in newtons per metre

☐   E   For a spherical shape, Laplace's law states that pressure gradient across the wall of a sphere is equal to $2 \times$ tension divided by the radius

2.58   Answers:

- A   True
- B   False
- C   False
- D   True
- E   True

Breathing air decreases turbulence as opposed to oxygen : nitrous oxide mix.

Tension is measured in newtons per metre acting on the length of a wall of tubing.

The critical flow rate is the rate of fluid/gas flow above which turbulence predominates, eg a 9-mm internal diameter ET tube has a critical flow rate of 9 l/min, above which the flow will become turbulent.

Although humidification increases the risk of turbulence, the predominant effect of humidification is a reduction in the turbulence secondary to the warming effect.

As gases are warmed by the time they reach the lower airways and as the flow is usually slower, laminar flow predominates.

Laplace's law for a tube is:

$P = T \div R$

where P is the pressure gradient across the wall, R is the radius and T is the tension.

Laplace's law for a sphere states: $P = 2T \div R$.

2.59 Regarding viscosity:

☐ A Blood viscosity increases with hypothermia

☐ B Viscosity is force per unit surface area divided by velocity gradient between adjacent fluid layers

☐ C Blood viscosity increases lineally with increasing haematocrit

☐ D Relative viscosity of normal plasma is 1.1

☐ E Relative viscosity of blood is 3.5

2.60 The following statements regarding fluid flow are correct:

☐ A A tube with a constriction with a cross-section that gradually decreases and then increases is known as a Venturi tube

☐ B Venturi refers to the fall in pressure at a constriction

☐ C At a constriction the kinetic energy of a fluid increases

☐ D Jet entrainment is caused by frictional forces

☐ E The entrainment ratio is defined as the ratio of driving flow divided by entrained flow

2.59 Answers:

- A True
- B True
- C False
- D False
- E True

Viscosity (measured in poise) is represented by the symbol η.

With increase in temperature the viscosity of blood falls.

With decrease in temperature the viscosity of blood rises.

Blood viscosity and haematocrit have a non-linear relationship.

As haematocrit increases blood viscosity increases exponentially.

Relative viscosity (ie when compared with water) of plasma is 1.5 and of normal whole blood 3.5.

2.60 Answers:

- A True
- B False
- C True
- D True
- E False

The fall in pressure at a constriction is known as the Bernoulli effect.

At a constriction the kinetic energy increases and, as total energy must remain the same (energy cannot be created or destroyed), the pressure or potential energy therefore decreases.

This causes the entrainment of fluid.

Jet entrainment refers to frictional forces that also increase the amount of fluid drawn into a system.

The entrainment ratio is defined as the ratio of entrained flow to driving flow.

2.61   Regarding the coanda effect:

☐   A   It was an effect originally applied to develop jet engines

☐   B   It refers to the adherence of fluid flow to a solid surface

☐   C   It may explain myocardial infarction in patients with patent vessels

☐   D   It can be used in ventilation

☐   E   A continuous jet of fluid across the nozzle is required to maintain flow down one limb

2.61   Answers:

- A True
- B True
- C True
- D True
- E False

At a point of constriction the pressure of fluid in a system falls.

If at this point the fluid is touching a wall, then nothing can be entrained as the negative pressure is spent holding the stream adjacent to that wall.

To change the flow of this fluid a jet of fluid can dislodge it to another wall.

The jet need not be continuous.

It can stop as soon as the flow of fluid has changed.

2.62   Regarding lung volumes and flow meters:

☐   A   Benedict Roth spirometers are accurate even at high respiratory rate

☐   B   The water seal of a Benedict Roth spirometer is large to prevent gas escaping from the system

☐   C   Vitalographs can be used to measure peak expiratory flow rate

☐   D   Vitalographs are suitable for measuring limited gas volumes

☐   E   The recording paper on a vitalograph is directly moved by the patient's respiratory efforts

2.62   Answers:

- A   False
- B   False
- C   True
- D   True
- E   False

Benedict Roth spirometers consist of a lightweight cylinder suspended over a breathing chamber with a water seal.

Vertical displacement of the cylinder is detected and recorded by a pen on a rotating drum.

The water seal is kept as small as possible to decrease the amount of gas absorbed.

At high respiratory rates inertia of the fluid in the system leads to inaccuracies.

Vitalographs and Benedict Roth spirometers are both suitable for measuring limited volumes, eg a few litres.

If larger volumes need to be measured other apparatus, eg dry gas meters, must be used.

The paper on a vitalograph is moved by a motor triggered by a patient's expiration.

The expiratory effort does not move the pen directly, otherwise this would present resistance to expiration.

2.63   Wright respirometers:

☐ A Can be used to measure continuous flow

☐ B Overestimate high volumes

☐ C Measure flow in one direction only

☐ D Are variable orifice flow meters

☐ E Measure flow in two directions

2.64   Regarding calculation of plasma volume and blood volume:

☐ A Plasma volume can be calculated according to the equation: plasma volume = (blood volume) ÷ (1 − haematocrit)

☐ B Radioactively labelled albumin is used to calculate plasma volume

☐ C Radioactively labelled sodium is used to measure total extracellular volume

☐ D The total amount of haemoglobin in a reservoir of 19 l of fluid with a concentration of haemoglobin of 3.5 g/l is approximately 5.4 g

☐ E The volume of blood lost = the amount of haemoglobin divided by concentration of haemoglobin

2.63   Answers:

- A   False
- B   True
- C   True
- D   True
- E   False

A Wright respirometer (a turbine flow meter) cannot be used to measure continuous flow as its calibration in these conditions is inaccurate.

It measures flow in one direction.

The vanes do not rotate if the flow is reversed.

It records volumes (tidal or minute ventilation).

It is inaccurate at high and low flows secondary to inertia or resistance respectively.

A Wright anemometer or peak flow meter is a variable orifice flow meter measuring flow in one direction.

2.64   Answers:

- A   False
- B   True
- C   True
- D   False
- E   True

Plasma volume = (blood volume) $\times$ (1 – haematocrit).

The equation written in option A would give a plasma volume greater than total blood volume, which clearly cannot be.

If 19 l of fluid have a haemoglobin concentration of 3.5 g/l, then the amount of haemoglobin present = 19 l $\times$ 3.5 g/l, which is 66.5 g.

The volume of blood lost:

= the amount of haemoglobin $\div$ concentration of haemoglobin

or the red cell volume $\div$ haematocrit

2.65 Regarding rotameters:

☐ A A constant pressure is present across the bobbin at all times

☐ B At low flows the viscosity of the gas is important

☐ C At high flows the viscosity of the gas is important

☐ D They are accurate within ± 0.2%

☐ E Although not ideal, oxygen and nitrous oxide rotameters can be interchanged as the gases have similar densities and viscosities

2.66 Regarding flow meters:

☐ A Oxygen flow meters are placed to the far left of the range of flow meters purely for historical reasons

☐ B Oxygen is added to the gas mixture last to prevent hypoxic gas mixture administration

☐ C Chain linking connects nitrous oxide and oxygen flow meters to prevent oxygen mixtures of less than 21% being administered

☐ D Gas flow meters on anaesthetic machines are positioned the same world-wide

☐ E A needle valve controls the flow into a rotameter

2.65   Answers:

- A   True
- B   True
- C   False
- D   False
- E   False

Rotameters are constant pressure, variable orifice, flow meters.

At low flows, laminar flow predominates.

Therefore viscosity is most important.

At high flows, the tube walls are a distance from the bobbin, so it acts as an orifice and turbulent flows predominate.

They are accurate to 2%.

Rotameters are individually calibrated according to the gas to be used and they are not interchangeable.

Nitrous oxide and carbon dioxide are two gases that are the closest in relation to their viscosity and density.

Nitrous oxide and oxygen rotameters certainly cannot be interchanged.

2.66   Answers:

- A   True
- B   True
- C   False
- D   False
- E   True

Boyle was left handed and therefore oxygen has historically been placed on the left on an anaesthetic machine; however, this is not the same world-wide.

In North America, the position of oxygen and nitrous oxide has been reversed so that a hypoxic mix secondary to a crack in the flow meter cannot be administered.

The lowest oxygen concentration delivered is 25% not 21%

2.67   Regarding pneumotachograph characteristics:

☐ A   They measure flow bi-directionally

☐ B   They have a variable orifice

☐ C   Gas flow is turbulent

☐ D   They are maintained at room temperature

☐ E   Integration of the flow can be used to record volume

2.68   Regarding flow meters:

☐ A   Bubble flow meters are useful for reading low flows

☐ B   Bubble flow meters are constant pressure variable orifices

☐ C   Heidbrink flow meters have a rotating bobbin indicator

☐ D   Watersight flow meters are constant pressure constant orifices

☐ E   Thermistor flow meters are reliant upon the cooling effect of a gas stream

2.67   Answers:
- A   True
- B   False
- C   False
- D   False
- E   True

A pneumotachograph is a constant orifice, variable pressure, flow meter.

It consists of an area of fixed resistance with pressure transducers on either side.

As the resistance is constant the pressure difference is a reflection of flow.

Flow is laminar not turbulent and therefore viscosity of the gas is important.

The presence of water is also important and, because of this, the pneumotachograph is heated.

2.68   Answers:
- A   True
- B   False
- C   False
- D   False
- E   True

To categorise flow meters:
- Constant orifice, variable pressure, eg pneumotachograph, water depression flow meters (simple water manometers).
- Variable orifice, constant pressure, eg rotameters, Heidbrink flow meter (the bobbin is non-rotating and rod shaped) and Wright respirometer.
- Variable orifice, variable pressure, eg watersight flow meter (gas passes through a tube with holes that is immersed in water).
- Constant orifice, constant pressure, eg bubble flow meter (gas passes through a tube with a soap film in it).
- Others including thermistors and ultrasonic flow meters.

Reference: Yentis SM. *Anaesthesia and Intensive Care A–Z*. 3rd edn. Butterworth–Heinemann, 2004.

2.69   Regarding intravenous infusion devices:

☐   A   Drip counters should be placed halfway between the drip-forming orifice and the liquid level

☐   B   The liquid in a drip counter chamber should occupy one-third of the space

☐   C   When the weight of a drip overcomes surface tension the drip will fall

☐   D   Temperature does not affect the drop size

☐   E   Drop size is uniform independent of fluid composition

2.70   The following statements regarding biological potentials are correct:

☐   A   The exterior of a nerve has a net positive charge of 90 mV compared with the interior

☐   B   Cardiac muscle remains depolarised for longer than skeletal muscle

☐   C   The size of the detected electrocardiogram (ECG) signal is 1–3 µV

☐   D   P-waves are usually positive despite the position of the ECG electrode as they spread outwards

☐   E   A normal PR interval is 0.12–0.2 seconds

2.69 Answers:

- A True
- B True
- C True
- D False
- E False

Drip counters are reliant upon a light-emitting diode and photo detection.

Drop size is variable with up to 20% variation and depends upon a number of variables, including density, surface tension, temperature and composition of the fluid.

Accurate drip counters are particularly important in paediatric fluid management.

2.70 Answers:

- A True
- B True
- C False
- D True
- E True

Cardiac muscle depolarisation is lengthened secondary to the influence of calcium ions.

The size of detected ECG signal is 1–2 mV not μV.

2.71   Electromyogram (EMG) potentials:

☐ A Range from 1 μV to 100 μV

☐ B Can be used for estimating depth of anaesthesia

☐ C Have a longer duration than ECG potentials

☐ D Have amplitude that is dependent upon the number of muscle fibres stimulated

☐ E Depolarise skeletal muscle in synchrony

2.72   Regarding electroencephalograph (EEG) potentials:

☐ A They range from 1 μV to 100 μV

☐ B α waves have the highest frequency

☐ C β activity decreases as age increases

☐ D α rhythms increase during general anaesthesia

☐ E δ waves have the lowest frequency

2.71 Answers:

- A False
- B True
- C False
- D True
- E False

EMG potentials range from approximately 10–100 µV to 10–100 mV.

They may be helpful as regards assessment of depth of anaesthesia when used to determine frontalis muscle tone.

EMG duration is shorter than that of the ECG secondary to the fact that skeletal muscle repolarises more quickly and skeletal muscle does not depolarise synchronously with adjacent cells.

2.72 Answers:

- A True
- B False
- C True
- D False
- E True

An EEG is a recording of electrical activity from the brain.

EEG potentials range from 1 µV to 100 µV.

Four waves are produced δ, θ, α and β in order of increasing frequency in hertz (Hz).

α waves are normal and prominent in the parieto-occipital area at rest and become depressed during anaesthesia.

β waves are prominent over the frontal area.

δ waves are normal in children and during sleep, otherwise they are abnormal.

θ waves can sometimes be abnormal.

Reference: Yentis SM. *Anaesthesia and Intensive Care A–Z*. 3rd edn. Butterworth–Heinemann, 2004.

2.73 When recording biological potentials:

☐ A Auditory evoked potentials are one of the first potentials to disappear as the depth of anaesthesia increases

☐ B Auditory evoked potentials can be recorded from electrodes attached to the mastoid and forehead

☐ C Compressed spectral array displays consecutive sections of EEGs as a series of peaks and troughs

☐ D Compressed spectral array requires EEG amplitude to be recorded

☐ E The bispectral index uses EEG analysis and phased coupling to produce a numerical value

2.74 Electrodes:

☐ A Can experience polarisation that can lead to inaccuracies in a detected signal

☐ B With silver chloride and chloride ions decrease inaccuracies by ensuring good skin contact

☐ C With a small surface area have reduced inaccuracies

☐ D Are unaffected by variable impedance at the skin

☐ E Can record inaccurate signals secondary to moisture at the point of skin and electrode contact

2.73   Answers:

- A   False
- B   True
- C   True
- D   True
- E   True

Auditory evoked potentials are one of the last potentials to disappear during anaesthesia and are therefore used as a measure of anaesthesia.

The forehead electrode is the reference electrode.

Compressed spectral array requires knowledge of the amplitude, time and frequency of EEG.

Bispectral index looks at the relationship between different frequency components, ie phased coupling together with other aspects of the EEG.

The bispectral index calculates a figure between 0 and 100, which is thought to give a guide to depth of anaesthesia.

2.74   Answers:

- A   True
- B   True
- C   False
- D   False
- E   True

When a signal arrives at an electrode, a small current is generated.

This can cause chemical changes at the surface of the electrode that can cause inaccuracies secondary to altered impedance.

This effect is polarisation.

Inaccuracies caused by electrodes resting on the skin also include impedance variation (eg moisture or electrode migration) and potential generation.

All of these inaccuracies are reduced by using silver electrodes in contact with its chloride ion in a gel solution.

2.75   Regarding amplifiers:

☐   A   The bandwidth of the amplifier enables rejection of some interference

☐   B   Differential amplifiers are not usually needed for EEG recordings

☐   C   Drift is more serious if an amplifier is designed only for AC potentials

☐   D   Temperature has minimal influence over drift

☐   E   The gain of an amplifier is measured on a logarithmic scale

2.75 Answers:

- A True
- B False
- C False
- D False
- E True

The bandwidth of the amplifier refers to the range of frequencies over which the amplifier is relatively constant.

If the current bandwidth is selected for the signal, then it can avoid some interference.

Differential amplifiers work on the principle of common mode rejection.

Only the difference in signal is recorded not the signal common to both.

This is crucial, particularly in EEG recording where the signal is so small that any interference will greatly distort the trace.

Drift is secondary to temperature changes causing a change in resistance in the semi-conductors used in amplifiers.

It causes DC potentials to change and is much less problematic with AC potentials.

In modern integrated circuits, the whole amplifier is formed on a very small silicon chip that does not allow any significant change in temperature to occur between the components.

The gain of the amplifier is the ratio of output voltage to input voltage and is measured in the unit called a bel.

Reference: *Anaesthesia and Intensive Care Medicine* 2005; 6: 301.

2.76   Regarding electrical potential generators:

☐   A   Inserted cardiac pacemakers have a pulse duration of less than 1 ms

☐   B   The negative electrode of a nerve simulator is placed over the nerve whereas the positive electrode is placed a few centimetres proximally

☐   C   The standard peripheral nerve stimulators used to assess neuromuscular function in theatre are set to deliver a maximum current of 60 mA

☐   D   Double-burst stimulation on a nerve stimulator produces two stimulations of 50 Hz for 60 ms

☐   E   Train-of-four stimulation delivers four stimuli at a rate of 4 Hz

2.76   Answers:

- A   True
- B   True
- C   True
- D   True
- E   False

The pulse duration of a pacemaker is less than 1 ms and the delivered potential can be as high as 4 V.

The negative electrode of a nerve stimulator is placed over the nerve with the positive electrode placed slightly more proximally.

The frequency of the pulse is dependent upon the test required by the nerve stimulator.

A dose of 60 mA is used for nerve stimulation as this is the supramaximal stimulus, ie 10–20% greater current than the threshold for the maximum stimulation.

In double-burst stimulation in option E, the stimuli are delivered 750 ms apart.

Train-of-four stimulation delivers four square-wave electrical pulses lasting 0.2 ms at a rate of 2 Hz.

2.77   TENS:

- ☐   A   Operates on the 'close the gate' principle
- ☐   B   Can be programmed to deliver currents as high as those used in a peripheral nerve stimulator, ie 60 mA
- ☐   C   Can lead to tissue damage
- ☐   D   Means the transcutaneous excitation of neuronal substances
- ☐   E   Aims to stimulate small afferent pain fibres

2.78   An oscilloscope (cathode ray tube):

- ☐   A   Relies upon the production of an ultraviolet beam
- ☐   B   Is particularly useful for displaying high-frequency signals
- ☐   C   Can be used to monitor arterial blood pressure from a transducer
- ☐   D   May be used to plot flow–volume loops
- ☐   E   Has an advantage over the galvanometer recorders as it has negligible inertia

2.77   Answers:

- A   True
- B   True
- C   True
- D   False
- E   False

TENS stands for transcutaneous electrical nerve stimulation and it is thought to be effective by stimulating large afferent fibres so that small afferent pain fibres transmitting chronic pain are inhibited.

Pulse duration is between 60 and 380 µs with a pulse frequency of 2–200 Hz.

Patients should be able to feel warmth and tingling while the TENS is working.

2.78   Answers:

- A   False
- B   True
- C   True
- D   True
- E   True

The cathode ray tube is used in medical monitoring including ECG and arterial blood pressure.

An oscilloscope relies on the production of an electron beam from a hot cathode, which is then acted upon by deflecting devices in both horizontal and vertical directions.

The sawtooth potential deflects the beam in a horizontal direction, whereas the biological potential to be monitored deflects it in a vertical direction.

As the oscilloscope has very little inertia (as opposed to the galvanometer recorders) it therefore has a very high-frequency response.

The electron beam is acted upon in both directions and accelerated and then displayed on a screen.

Two signals can be plotted at once so flow–volume loops can be recorded.

2.79   Regarding the principles of magnetism and magnetic flux:

☐ A There must be a current flow through iron alloy for magnetism to occur

☐ B Magnetic flux decreases the power of the magnetic field in a vacuum

☐ C If a conductor is placed into a coil a current flowing in it produces a magnetic field, which is strongest within the core of the coil

☐ D Magnetic flux is measured in magnons

☐ E Magnetic flux density is measured in teslas

2.80   Regarding magnetic flux:

☐ A It is measured in webers

☐ B 1 tesla = 1 weber per square metre

☐ C Magnetic flux density in air is approximately 60 teslas

☐ D It is greater than magnetic field strength in diamagnetic materials

☐ E It is slightly greater than magnetic field strength in paramagnetic materials

2.79   Answers:

- A True
- B False
- C True
- D False
- E True

Although iron alloy may appear to be magnetic without any obvious current flowing within it, many small currents formed by the movement of electrons orbiting around the nuclei can cause magnetism without obvious current flow.

Magnetic flux describes the field formed which results when a magnetic field is present in a piece of material, whereas magnetic field strength describes the power of the field in a vacuum.

Magnetic flux is measured in units of webers, whereas magnetic flux density is measured in teslas.

2.80   Answers:

- A True
- B True
- C False
- D False
- E True

Magnetic flux (measured in webers) describes the field resulting when a magnetic field is present is any material.

Magnetic flux density, measured in teslas, is the magnetic flux divided by the area in square metres.

Permanent magnets can possess a magnetic flux density of 1 tesla (T).

MRI scanners have a magnetic flux density of 0.1–4 T.

Earths magnetic field produces a magnetic flux density of approximately 60 μT.

Magnetic flux is increased greatly when compared with magnetic field strength in ferromagnetic materials.

It is increased slightly in paramagnetic materials and decreased in diamagnetic materials.

2.81   Regarding direct and alternating currents:

☐   A   The base SI unit of current is the ampere

☐   B   One ampere represents flow of 6.18×10^{24} electrons per second past some point

☐   C   The following statement is correct: a wire carrying electrical current in a magnetic field creates a force that moves in a direction perpendicular to both the electric current and the magnetic field

☐   D   Thermocouples are a source of direct current

☐   E   Rechargeable batteries are able to supply alternating current

2.82   Regarding electricity:

☐   A   It can be used to measure blood flow in the form of electromagnetism

☐   B   Power equivalent of 12 W with a current flow of 6 A will give a potential difference of 2 V

☐   C   Root mean square values are used commercially

☐   D   The peak voltage of mains potential in the UK is 240 V

☐   E   To obtain an equivalent direct current (DC) value, alternating current (AC) values must be squared, then averaged, then rooted

2.81 Answers:

- A True
- B False
- C True
- D True
- E False

The base SI unit of current is the ampere, which represents flow of 6.24×10^{18} electrons per second past some point or the current that produces a force of 2×10^{-7} N/m between two conductors, 1 m apart in a vacuum.

Galvanometers are reliant upon the principle in option C.

Rechargeable batteries supply direct current.

To recharge, current is passed into the battery in the reverse direction to the flow of current out of the battery.

This reverses the chemical reaction and enables the battery to be used again.

2.82 Answers:

- A True
- B True
- C True
- D False
- E True

Electromagnetic flow meters are used to measure blood flow.

Movement of a conductor through a magnetic field produces an electrical potential the size of which is dependent upon the rate of movement of the conductor.

Blood is able to conduct electricity and can therefore be measured by this technique.

Potential differences in volts = power in watts divided by current in amperes ($V = P \div I$); therefore $12 \div 6 = 2$.

Root mean square values are used commercially, so mains voltage at 240 V is actually its root mean square value.

To calculate the root mean square value the AC value must be squared, then averaged and then rooted (see option E).

The peak voltage of the mains supply is actually 340 V.

2.83   When using diathermy:

☐ A The risk of VF (ventricular fibrillation) decreases as the current frequency increases

☐ B It utilises the theory of current density

☐ C It has a frequency of approximately 100 MHz

☐ D Poor plate position can lead to burns with bipolar diathermy

☐ E All forms of diathermy can operate at high powers

2.83   Answers:

- A True
- B True
- C True
- D False
- E False

The risk of VF increases with a decrease in current frequency.

Diathermy works on the principle that a high-frequency current is passed through tissue to cause cutting and coagulation.

The smaller the contact with the tissue, the higher the current density and the greater the diathermy effect.

Bipolar diathermy does not require a patient plate.

Electrical current passes down one pair of forceps and into the other without passing through the body.

The disadvantage of bipolar diathermy is that it cannot operate at high powers.

2.84   Regarding electrical components:

☐ A Transformers rely upon induction of current from one coil to
            another

☐ B Diodes transmit only alternating current

☐ C Transistors convert one type of energy into another

☐ D The equation $V_2 = V_1 \times (n_1 \div n_2)$, where V = voltage and n is
            the number of coils relied upon when referring to amplifiers

☐ E A rectangular box in a line is the symbol for a resistor

2.84   Answers:

- A   True
- B   False
- C   False
- D   False
- E   True

Transformers are composed of two inductors wound around the same form.

The two coils of inductors are positioned close together such that a current in coil number 1 will induce a current in coil number 2 by the coupling effect of the magnetic field as per the equation: $V_2 = V_1 \times (n_2 \div n_1)$.

Transformers can be used to either step up or step down currents.

Diodes allow current flow in one direction only, ie only direct current flows.

Transducers convert one type of energy into another.

Transistors allow passage of current; when a small current is applied to the base they can be used to amplify a signal.

The symbol for a resistor is:

–▢–

2.85   Regarding capacitance and charge:

☐ A Capacitance is the measure of the ability to hold an electric charge

☐ B Capacitance is measured in coulombs (C)

☐ C One unit of charge is the amount of electricity equivalent to 6.24×10^{18} electrons

☐ D Charge is equal to capacitance divided by voltage

☐ E A capacitor is composed of two insulting plates separated by a conductor

2.85   Answers:

- A True
- B False
- C True
- D False
- E False

Capacitance is measured in farad (F).

A capacitor has 1 F of capacitance if 1 V is the potential difference across its plates when a charge of 1 C is held by the plates.

Coulombs are the unit of charge.

$C = F \times V$, where F = capacitance in farads, C = charge in coulombs and V = potential difference in volts.

A capacitor has two conducting plates separated by an insulator.

The insulator is known as the dielectric.

Reference: *Anaesthesia and Intensive Care Medicine* 2005; 6: 298.

2.86 Defibrillators:

☐ A Rely on direct current

☐ B Have a potential difference between the plates of their capacitor of up to 5000 V

☐ C Operate on the principle that stored energy = stored charge × potential

☐ D Have circuits containing an inductor to increase the peak energy delivered

☐ E Should be synchronised with the R-wave when cardioverting ventricular tachycardia with a pulse

2.86   Answers:

- A   True
- B   True
- C   False
- D   False
- E   True

A defibrillator circuit consists of a capacitor, a number of switches and an inductor.

Up to 5000 V are applied across the capacitor producing a store of electrons equivalent to 160 mC of charge.

Stored energy = 0.5 × stored charge × potential.

Once discharged current flows initially through an inductor and then through paddles to the patient's chest.

The inductor acts to smooth out the flow of current.

The current does not flow immediately but slowly increases as magnetic force increases.

When the voltage is stopped the current gradually dies down.

It therefore optimises electrical pulse shape and duration.

2.87   Regarding electricity:

☐ A No current will flow when direct current is applied to an
        uncharged capacitor

☐ B Capacitance can be the cause of electrical interference on an
        ECG trace

☐ C Inductance can be the cause of electrical interference on an
        ECG trace

☐ D An inductor is typically a coil of wire

☐ E Screening involves reducing interference by insulating the
        wires with plastic

2.88   Regarding signal-to-noise ratio:

☐ A Noise from capacitance and inductance can be reduced with
        differential amplifiers

☐ B A high signal-to-noise ratio is desirable

☐ C It can be improved by amplification of the waveform

☐ D It will not be improved by averaging a repetitive waveform

☐ E Electronic filters designed to filter low-frequency signals are
        used to reduce interference from diathermy

2.87   Answers:

- A   False
- B   True
- C   True
- D   True
- E   False

If direct current is passed through an uncharged capacitor, current will flow initially until the capacitor plate becomes charged, at which point no further current will flow.

Both capacitance and inductance can lead to interference.

An inductor is a coil of wire with a ferrous magnetic core.

It is part of the working of a defibrillator.

Screening is a process of interference reduction by covering monitoring leads with a sheath of earthed woven metal so that interference currents are induced in this rather than in the monitoring leads.

2.88   Answers:

- A   True
- B   True
- C   False
- D   False
- E   False

Amplification of the signal also amplifies noise and is therefore unhelpful.

Averaging a repetitive waveform is, however, helpful.

Noise will be averaged to zero, as it is random in nature, whereas the signal will remain constant.

Diathermy interference is reduced by the presence of a high-frequency electronic filter not a low-frequency one.

2.89   Regarding resistance:

☐ A The ohm is the base SI unit

☐ B The resistance of a wire increases with temperature

☐ C The resistance of a wire decreases with stretching

☐ D Ohm's law states that: resistance = potential (volts) ÷ current (amps)

☐ E A Wheatstone bridge circuit needs only four resistors and a galvanometer to function

2.90   Regarding the resistance to current flow:

☐ A The resistance of a resistor to alternating current varies with the frequency of the current

☐ B Capacitors allow high-frequency current to flow more easily than low frequency

☐ C Inductors allow high-frequency current through more easily than low frequency

☐ D The unit of impedance is the same as that of capacitance

☐ E The term 'impedance' is used when there is a difference in current flow dependent upon the frequency of the current

2.89   Answers:

- A False
- B True
- C False
- D True
- E False

The ohm is a derived SI unit of resistance but it is not a base SI unit.

There are only seven base SI units: candela, mole, second, metre, kilogram, ampere and kelvin.

Stretching a wire makes it thinner and therefore increases its resistance.

A Wheatstone bridge circuit needs four resistors (R_1–R_4), a galvanometer and a source of electrical potential.

One resistor (R_4) can be a strain gauge transducer or a resistance thermometer and one resistor (R_3) can be of variable resistance so that it can be adjusted to give a galvanometer reading of zero.

On this basis: $R_1 \div R_2 = R_3 \div R_4$

2.90   Answers:

- A False
- B True
- C False
- D False
- E True

The resistance of a resistor is unaffected by the current frequency.

Inductors are opposite to capacitors and allow low-frequency currents to pass preferentially.

The unit of impedance is the ohm and this is the same as the unit of resistance; however, it takes the symbol Z.

The farad (F) is the unit of capacitance.

2.91   Regarding impedance:

☐ A Skin impedance reduces with moisture

☐ B It is reduced if good contact is made with skin and the ECG electrode

☐ C Electrode gel on ECG electrodes predominantly reduces the skin impedance

☐ D Amplifiers with high-input impedance are used with electrodes now to give negligible attenuation of the input signal

☐ E Galvanic skin response is dependent on skin impedance recordings

2.92   The following are true of waves and wavelengths:

☐ A The phase of a sine wave refers to the different speed at which the wave crosses the horizontal line

☐ B The wavelength of a sine wave is the distance from the horizontal line to the peak of the wave

☐ C A large amplitude light wave produces a dim light

☐ D Hertz is the unit that denotes frequency

☐ E The period of wave motion (ie the time taken for one complete cycle to occur) is the reciprocal of the frequency

2.91 Answers:

- A True
- B True
- C False
- D True
- E True

The gel surrounding electrodes is predominantly to reduce electrical impedance not skin impedance.

The galvanic skin response is a test performed whereby the autonomic activity of the patient can be monitored secondary to the change in the skin impedance.

With activation of the sympathetic nerve system the skin becomes moist and therefore the skin impedance falls.

2.92 Answers:

- A False
- B False
- C False
- D True
- E True

The phase of a sine wave refers to the different angles that the wave crosses the horizontal line.

It is described in degrees.

Option B refers to the amplitude of the wave whereas the wavelength is the distance between any two corresponding points in successive cycles.

Large amplitude light waves produce bright light.

Hertz is the unit for cycles per second and is the derived SI unit of frequency.

If the period of the wave motion = T, then $T = 1 \div$ frequency (in Hz)

2.93   Regarding waves and wavelengths:

☐ A   Velocity = frequency ÷ wavelength

☐ B   Sound has a velocity of 330 m/s in air

☐ C   Short wavelengths have high frequencies (presuming that velocity is kept constant)

☐ D   Radiowaves have a higher frequency than X-rays

☐ E   Sounds with a low frequency sound low pitched

2.94   Regarding the electromagnetic spectrum:

☐ A   Paging systems have a long wavelength when compared with X-rays

☐ B   Ultraviolet and visible waves are quoted as a unit of energy called the electronvolt (eV)

☐ C   X-rays and γ waves used clinically have energy ranges from kilo-electronvolts to mega-electronvolts

☐ D   Velocity of the electromagnetic spectrum is significantly reduced in air compared with a vacuum

☐ E   Radar waves have a higher frequency than γ rays

2.93   Answers:

- A False
- B True
- C True
- D False
- E True

Velocity = frequency × wavelength. ie $V = f\lambda$.

If velocity (V) is constant, as wavelength (λ) decreases, frequency (f) increases.

Red light has a low frequency and longer wavelength compared with blue light.

Radiowaves have a low frequency (audible) compared with X-rays.

2.94   Answers:

- A True
- B False
- C True
- D False
- E False

The electromagnetic spectrum is made up of a range of different waveforms.

They all have the same velocity in a vacuum: 3×10^8 m/s.

The waves vary according to their wavelength and frequency, with low frequency accompanying long wavelength.

Their velocity is not significantly affected by air but they are markedly slowed by liquid and solid interfaces.

X-rays and γ waves are quoted in electronvolts (eV) whereas UV and visible waves are quoted as wavelengths of micrometres or nanometres.

Waves in order of increasing frequency or decreasing wavelength are radiowaves, infrared, visible, UV and X-rays and γ waves.

2.95   Regarding the Doppler effect:

☐ A   As the signal source approaches the observer, the observed frequency of the signal increases

☐ B   It detects the change in frequency of a returning sound wave

☐ C   It can be used as an indicator of cardiac output

☐ D   As a sound source moves towards a listener the wavelength increases

☐ E   The frequency of ultrasound is so low that we are unable to hear it

2.96   Regarding density:

☐ A   Density is measured in grams per litre

☐ B   Specific gravity is the ratio of the density of a substance to a standard

☐ C   Baricity is a measure of a ratio

☐ D   Density is unaffected by temperature

☐ E   The mean density of cerebrospinal fluid (CSF) is less than that of interstitial fluid

2.95   Answers:

- A True
- B True
- C True
- D False
- E False

As a sound source moves towards an observer the velocity is unchanged, so the wavelength and frequency vary inversely.

The wavelength decreases and the frequency increases, so the sound becomes higher pitched.

Ultrasound emits a very high-frequency, low-wavelength signal, which is too high to be audible to the human ear.

2.96   Answers:

- A True
- B True
- C True
- D False
- E False

When using the example of CSF with a mean density of 1.0003 g/l it is measured at 37°C.

Temperature affects density and therefore must be specified.

Baricity is analogous to specific density but, whereas specific gravity is the ratio of density of a substance to a standard, baricity is the ratio of the density of a substance compared with another substance at a specific temperature.

Mean density of CSF is very similar to that of interstitial fluid.

Reference: Intrathecal drug spread. *British Journal of Anaesthesia* 2004; 93(4): 568–78.

2.97   Regarding a pulmonary artery flotation catheter:

☐ A It is 70 cm long

☐ B The proximal port is 12 cm from the tip

☐ C The introducer sheath is 10 G

☐ D The distance from the proximal injectate port to the thermistor
            is 5 cm

☐ E The balloon should be inflated with 2.5 ml air

2.97   Answers:

- A True
- B False
- C False
- D False
- E False

The average pulmonary artery flotation catheter is 70 cm long with a distal port at the tip.

The thermistor is a few centimetres from the tip.

The proximal port is 30 cm from the tip.

Around 1–1.5 ml air should be used to inflate the balloon.

The introducer sheath is 8 G.

2.98   **When referring to blood gas analysis:**

☐   A   The actual base excess is the absolute difference in buffer base from the normal amount in blood.

☐   B   The standard base excess cBase (Ecf) is an estimate more representative of an in vivo base excess than the actual base excess cBase (a)

☐   C   Actual bicarbonate is measured by the analyser

☐   D   The standard bicarbonate eliminates any effect that CO_2 in the sample has on the result

☐   E   The reference range for standard bicarbonate is higher than that for actual bicarbonate

2.98   Answers:

- A   True
- B   True
- C   False
- D   True
- E   False

Actual base excess with the definition cBase (A) is the concentration of titratable base (comprising bicarbonate, haemoglobin, plasma proteins and phosphate) when the sample is mixed with a strong acid or base to achieve a plasma pH of 7.4 at a $PaCO_2$) of 5.3 kPa at 37°C.

Whereas the actual base excess represents the total buffering capacity of blood, the standard base excess calculates the base excess according to extracellular fluid-buffering capacity alone.

It assumes a standard value for the haemoglobin concentration of the total extracellular fluid (including blood) of 3 mmol/l.

The result is a more accurate representation of in vivo base excess.

Bicarbonate is not measured; it is calculated according to the measured pH and PCO_2 values.

The actual bicarbonate is calculated according to the Henderson–Hasselbalch equation.

The standard bicarbonate is the concentration of hydrogen carbonate in plasma once it has been equilibrated at PCO_2 5.3 kPa and PO_2 13.3 kPa at 37°C.

This eliminates any respiratory function bias on the bicarbonate result.

The reference range for standard bicarbonate in men is 22.5–26.9 mmol/l compared with actual bicarbonate range of 24–31 mmol/l.

2.99   Heat loss in adults in normal situations:

☐   A   Is predominantly secondary to radiation

☐   B   Is greater by convection than evaporation

☐   C   By conduction is significant

☐   D   As a result of respiration is predominantly secondary to warming of the inspired air

☐   E   By evaporation can increase 10-fold by sweating

2.99   Answers:

- A   True
- B   True
- C   False
- D   False
- E   True

The typical forms of heat loss are shown in the table below.

Type of heat loss	Percentage contribution
Radiation	40
Convection	30
Evaporation	20
Respiration	10

Radiation may account for over 40% of heat loss.

It is secondary to the transfer of predominantly infrared radiation from a hot object to another less hot one.

These two objects do not need to be in contact and the extent of infrared radiation transfer depends on the characteristics and temperatures of the exchanging objects.

Radiation in theatre is reduced with shiny metallised reflective caps.

These cannot be safely used as body covers in theatre because they pose a burns and electric shock risk.

Convection is reduced in theatre by warm air blowers.

Respiration accounts for only a small percentage of heat loss.

It results predominantly from humidification of the inspired gas (80%), not warming (only 20%).

2.100 The following are correct regarding safety precautions when using lasers:

☐ A All personnel must wear protective skin garments

☐ B Carbon dioxide lasers cause most damage to the retina

☐ C Goggles that protect against carbon dioxide lasers will be suitable for most other laser types

☐ D High-energy laser beams are not able to ignite rubber

☐ E Helium should be avoided

2.100 Answers:

- A False
- B False
- C False
- D False
- E False

The skin of the patient should be protected but it is unnecessary for personnel to be covered.

The ocular risk for personnel is because of direct shining of the laser or reflection of a shiny surface, eg surgical instruments.

Carbon dioxide lasers have a long wavelength (10 600 nm) and are absorbed in 200 μm of tissue, so the cornea is most at risk.

Other lasers are focused by the lens onto the retina, causing damage in a short period.

Infrared light is particularly dangerous as it is not in the visible spectrum and causes damage to the cornea, lens, and aqueous and vitreous humours.

Most goggles absorb carbon dioxide laser beams but special goggles are required for other lasers.

Metallic or metallic coated tubes are used as rubber, PVC and silicone tubes are liable to ignite.

Helium and nitrogen are inert and are therefore advised.

Reference: Lasers and surgery. *British Journal of Anaesthesia CEPD Reviews* 2003; 3(5): 143–6.

2.101 High airflow oxygen enrichment (HAFOE) devices:

☐ A Work on the Bernoulli effect

☐ B Entrain oxygen

☐ C Rely on the peak inspiratory flow rate being ⩽ 30 l/min

☐ D An oxygen flow rate of 8 l/min is needed for an inspired oxygen concentration of 40%

☐ E The highest inspired oxygen concentration is 75%

2.102 Regarding humidification devices:

☐ A Cold water bubble-through is more efficient than heat and moisture exchanger

☐ B A heated water bath is more efficient than a heat and moisture exchanger

☐ C A heated water baths are normally heated to 40–45°C

☐ D A heated Bernoulli nebuliser with anvil is more efficient at humidification than ultrasonic nebulisers

☐ E Heat and moisture exchangers can give erroneously high airway pressure readings

2.101 Answers:

- A True
- B False
- C True
- D False
- E False

HAFOE devises work on the Venturi principle and the Bernoulli effect of entrainment of air not oxygen.

They deliver a predictable oxygen fraction according to the oxygen flow, based on the following equation:

$100a \times 21b = 30 \times$ required FiO_2

where $a =$ oxygen flow rate and $b =$ entrained airflow rate, provided that the peak inspiratory flow is not greater than 30 l/min.

The highest FiO_2 delivered is 60% with 15 l/min oxygen flow. With an oxygen rate of 8 l/min the delivered FiO_2 is 35% compared with 40% with 10 l/min oxygen.

2.102 Answers:

- A False
- B True
- C True
- D False
- E True

The following devices are ranked with the least efficient first: cold water bubble-through, heat and moisture exchange, heated water bath, heated Bernoulli nebuliser and anvil, and finally ultrasonic nebuliser.

Heated water baths are normally heated to 40–45°C; however, sometimes higher temperatures are used for prevention of bacterial growth.

Obviously appropriate precautions are employed to prevent risk of airway burns including a thermostat.

Heat and moisture exchangers must be changed regularly, as moisture accumulates and resistance greatly increases.

This result can lead to high airway pressure readings that are unrelated to the patient's ventilatory system.

2.103 The following are true regarding the cleansing of medical equipment:

☐ A Without standard precautions, hepatitis C can be transmitted via breathing circuits

☐ B Laryngoscopes are categorised as non-critical items according to the Spaulding classification of infection risk

☐ C Critical items, as identified by the Spaulding classification, must be sterile at the time of use

☐ D The cleaning process of cavitation involves ultrasonic cleaning

☐ E Cleaning is important to reduce the bioburden before disinfection or sterilisation

2.103 Answers:

- A True
- B False
- C True
- D True
- E True

Hepatitis C infection and resistant tuberculosis in anaesthetic breathing circuits lead to the introduction of single-use bacterial/ viral filters.

The Spaulding classification, devised in 1968, divides hospital equipment into three categories according to the infection risk to the patient.

Each category has a recommended level of decontamination:

Category	Definition and example	Recommended decontamination
Critical item	Enter sterile tissue or vascular system, eg surgical instruments/catheters	Sterilisation
Semi-critical item	In contact with mucosal membrane and non-intact skin Don't break blood barrier, eg laryngoscope, breathing circuits, fibreoptic endoscopes	At least high-level disinfection Cleaned at point of use
Non-critical item	In contact with healthy skin, eg blood pressure cuffs, pulse oximeters	

Cavitation is the process of the ultrasonic creation of tiny bubbles in a fluid-filled cleaning chamber.

The bubbles implode on the hard-to-reach crevices on equipment, creating a negative pressure that pulls the debris off.

Reference: Decontamination of anaesthetic equipment. *Continuing Education in Anaesthesia, Critical Care and Pain* 2004; 4(4): 103–6.

2.104 When cleaning medical equipment:

☐ A Pasteurisation is an example of disinfection

☐ B Alcohols (60–80%) will kill some viruses

☐ C Chemical incompatibility prevents chemical disinfection of certain devises

☐ D Bacterial spores are killed by pasteurisation for 30 minutes at 77°C

☐ E Postprocessing rinsing is essential after pasteurisation

2.104 Answers:

- A True
- B True
- C True
- D False
- E False

Pasteurisation is a method of disinfection that utilises hot water for different periods. It does not kill bacterial spores.

There is no risk of toxic postprocessing chemical residue, so rinsing is not required.

Alcohol is used as a low-level chemical disinfectant and will kill most vegetative bacteria and some viruses and fungi. It does not reduce spore activity.

Reference: Decontamination of anaesthetic equipment. *Continuing Education in Anaesthesia, Critical Care and Pain* 2004; 4(4): 103–6.

2.105 Sterilisation of medical equipment:

☐ A Is the process by which all types of micro-organisms including spores are killed

☐ B Using steam is the preferred method if the device can withstand it

☐ C Can be performed with glutaraldehyde 2%

☐ D Using ethylene oxide results from alkylation of proteins

☐ E By gas plasma can occur with a cycle time of less than 2 hours

2.105 Answers:

- A True
- B True
- C True
- D True
- E True

Steam sterilisation is efficient and safe.

If the device can withstand the temperatures required, it is the preferred method.

Chemical sterilisation using glutaraldehyde 2%, ethylene oxide or gas plasma can be used if steam sterilisation is unsuitable.

Glutaraldehyde and ethylene oxide sterilisation are lengthy processes requiring more than 10 hours and 2–12 hours respectively.

Gas plasma sterilisation results from highly ionised gas, containing ions and free radicals, diffusing through packaging and inactivating micro-organisms.

The process takes only 75 minutes.

Gamma irradiation is used commercially for sterilisation but is expensive and not the preferred method for hospital use.

Reference: Decontamination of anaesthetic equipment. *Continuing Education in Anaesthesia, Critical Care and Pain* 2004; 4(4): 103–6.

2.106 Awareness during anaesthesia:

☐ A Is not more likely to occur when using neuromuscular blockade

☐ B Is more likely during emergency surgery

☐ C May be more likely when using total intravenous anaesthesia (TIVA) because of the greater variation in dosing required

☐ D Is closely related to minimum alveolar concentration (MAC) values of exhaled volatile agent

☐ E Can be associated with impurities in the volatile agent

2.106 Answers:

- A False
- B True
- C True
- D True
- E True

Awareness can be in the form of explicit or implicit memory of events.

Explicit memory can be recalled with or without prompting.

Implicit memory cannot be consciously recalled but may still have detrimental effects on the behaviour of the individual.

There is a twofold increase in likelihood of awareness when using neuromuscular blockade.

Other situations associated with increased incidence of awareness include emergency and cardiac surgery and cases associated with hypotension, eg haemorrhage, where there is reluctance to decrease blood pressure further with vasodilating anaesthetics.

It is thought that the minimum inhibitory concentration (MIC) of intravenous anaesthetics has a larger variability compared with MAC.

This and the limitation of monitoring intravenous concentration of anaesthetics may lead to an increased incidence of awareness with TIVA.

In standard patients (and assuming that the end-tidal pressure equilibrates with brain partial pressure) with end-tidal volatile concentrations of >0.8 MAC, it is unlikely that they will experience intraoperative recall.

At levels >1 MAC, the risk of awareness in a standard patient is negligible.

Impurities in the volatile agent can decrease saturated vapour pressure and therefore decrease brain partial pressure.

Reference: Awareness during anaesthesia. *Continuing Education in Anaesthesia, Critical Care and Pain* 2005; 5(6): 183–6.

2.107 Regarding awareness:

- ☐ A Glycopyrrolate can mask the signs of sweating
- ☐ B Midazolam administration will provide reliable retrograde amnesia
- ☐ C Hypothermia is a risk factor
- ☐ D It is more likely in the obese patient
- ☐ E It is more likely in hyperbaric conditions

2.107 Answers:

- A True
- B False
- C False
- D True
- E False

A number of drugs can mask the sympathetic signs that may indicate awareness to noxious stimulus including glycopyrrolate and β-blockers.

Midazolam given preoperatively may reduce awareness; however, if awareness is suspected, it has not been proven to cause retrograde amnesia.

Situations that increase MAC may be associated with increased awareness including hypermetabolic states, chronic drug abuse and anxiety.

Hypothermia reduces MAC.

In a hyperbaric atmosphere, the sensitivity to anaesthetic agents is unaltered but the inspired and therefore the brain partial pressure are increased for a given inspired concentration.

Reference: Awareness during anaesthesia. *Continuing Education in Anaesthesia, Critical Care and Pain* 2005; 5(6): 183–6.

2.108 When monitoring depth of anaesthesia:

☐ A The isolated forearm technique may be appropriate for operations of long duration

☐ B Tear formation is a reliable indicator

☐ C The EEG reveals a decrease in frequency and amplitude as depth of anaesthesia increases

☐ D Burst suppression on EEG is not a reliable indicator

☐ E PRST scoring is a measure of stimulation of the sympathetic nervous system

2.108 Answers:

- A False
- B False
- C True
- D False
- E True

The isolated forearm technique is not commonly used.

It would be inappropriate for operations of long duration because of the tourniquet effect exerted by the pneumatic cuff.

Although tear formation may indicate sympathetic activity, sympathetic signs have not been shown to correlate well with incidence of awareness.

PRST scoring (systolic arterial **P**ressure, pulse **R**ate, **S**weating, **T**ear formation) is a measure of sympathetic stimulation.

Burst suppression on EEG is associated with deep anaesthesia.

2.109 The following use an EEG to monitor depth of anaesthesia:

☐ A Compressed spectral array

☐ B Auditory evoked potential

☐ C Bispectral index (BIS) technique

☐ D Frontalis muscle

☐ E Isolated forearm technique

2.110 Regarding filters:

☐ A Commonly used blood giving sets have a filter of 200 µm

☐ B Epidural filters are a 0.22-µm mesh

☐ C Platelets can be administered via a 200-µm filter

☐ D A standard filter needle has a 5-µm filter size

☐ E FFP can be given via a standard giving set

2.109 Answers:

- A True
- B True
- C True
- D False
- E False

Frontalis muscle contraction is measured by EMG.

Isolated forearm technique utilises movements observed by the operator.

Compressed spectral array is a process where EEG data are subject to Fourier transformation, giving a total power contained within different frequencies.

The BIS technique uses a different mathematical calculation to determine the relationship between frequencies on the EEG.

The BIS technique uses a combination of spectral array, bispectral analysis and burst suppression to give a measure of the depth of anaesthesia.

2.110 Answers:

- A True
- B True
- C True
- D True
- E True

Platelets can be administered via a standard giving set with a filter size of 200 μm (as marked on the giving set packaging) or via a platelet-giving set.

Platelets should not be transfused through a giving set that has been used for blood.

2.111 Regarding the use of fibres filtration:

☐ A Of large particles can be achieved by direct interception

☐ B By diffusion interception is because of constant random movement of particles

☐ C By electrostatic attraction is increased if the charge on the fibres is increased

☐ D By electrostatic filters has an efficiency of 99.99%

☐ E Results in reduced efficiency of electrostatic filters as they become wet

2.111 Answers:

- A True
- B True
- C True
- D True
- E True

There are five methods of filtration by fibres:

1. Direct interception occurs when particles (≥ 1 μm) are too large to pass.
2. Inertial impaction causes particles (0.5–1 μm) to collide with the fibres where they are held by van der Waals' forces.
3. Diffusion interception prevents passage of small particles (<0.5 μm) with small mass as the constant movement causes inevitable collision with the fibres.
4. Electrostatic attraction occurs as charged particles are attracted to the oppositely charged fibre.
5. Gravitation setting occurs as large particles (>5 μm) settle under the influence of gravity.

The electrostatic charge of filters decreases when wet.

2.112 Breathing systems: the following fresh gas flows (FGFs) are appropriate to prevent rebreathing:

☐ A 70 ml/kg per min when using a Mapleson A circuit in a spontaneously breathing patient

☐ B Alveolar minute volume in a ventilated patient when using a Mapleson B circuit

☐ C 70 ml/kg per min when using a Mapleson D circuit in a ventilated patient

☐ D 2–3 × minute volume when using a Mapleson E circuit in a spontaneously breathing patient

☐ E 70 ml/kg per min when using the Humphrey ADE system in a ventilated patient

2.112 Answers:

- A True
- B False
- C True
- D True
- E True

Mapleson breathing circuit	FGF in spontaneous breathing	FGF for ventilation
A	70 ml/kg per min	2–3 × minute volume
B	2–3 × minute volume	2–3 × minute volume
C	2–3 × minute volume	2–3 × minute volume
D	150–250 ml/kg per min	70 ml/kg per min (100 ml/kg per min for hypocapnia)
E	2–3 × minute volume	2–3 × minute volume
F	2–3 × minute volume	2–3 × minute volume
ADE	50–60 ml/kg per min	70 ml/kg per min

References: Aitkenhead A, Rowbottom D, Smith GA. *Textbook of Anaesthesia*. 4th edn. Churchill Livingstone, 2001.

Al-Shaikh B, Stacey S. *Essentials of Anaesthetic Equipment*, 2nd edn. Churchill Livingstone, 2001

2.113 Regarding anaesthetic breathing systems:

☐ A The minimum recommended flow on a Mapleson E circuit is 2 l/min

☐ B Efficient scavenging is a problem with Mapleson F circuits

☐ C Movement of the reservoir bag on a Bain circuit confirms delivery of fresh gas to the patient

☐ D A Manley ventilator set to spontaneous ventilation is an example of a non-coaxial Mapleson D

☐ E When ventilating with a Penlon via a Bain circuit, the corrugated tube that attaches the ventilator to the Bain can be of any volume

2.113 Answers:

- A False
- B True
- C False
- D True
- E False

The minimum recommended FGF on a Mapleson E circuit is 3–4 l/min.

At lower FGF, there is the risk of inhaling air at the end of inspiration if the patient's tidal volume is greater than the volume of the corrugated tube.

There is no standard efficient way of scavenging when using a Mapleson F circuit.

Movement of the reservoir bag on a Bain circuit indicates movement of gas but does not give indication of delivery of FGF to the patient.

It provides no warning of inner tube disconnection.

The volume of the corrugated tubing that attaches the ventilator to the Bain circuit is important, as too small a length will lead to ventilator-driving gas diluting the FGF.

The recommended volume is >500 ml.

2.114 Laryngoscopes:

☐ A The tip of a straight blade should be placed in the vallecula

☐ B The McCoy laryngoscope has a hinged blade tip

☐ C Straight blades are more likely to bruise the epiglottis than curved blades

☐ D Left-sided blades are for left-handed anaesthetists

☐ E Polio blades open to an angle of about 120°

2.115 The following are correct regarding pacemakers:

☐ A Letter position 2 refers to the chamber sensed

☐ B Letter position 4 refers to the antitachyarrhythmia function

☐ C Symptomatic second-degree heart block, regardless of the type, is an indication for a permanent pacemaker

☐ D Hypercapnia has no effect on the excitation threshold required to generate a contraction

☐ E Modern pacemakers are bipolar

2.114 Answers:

- A False
- B True
- C True
- D False
- E True

The standard curved Macintosh blade is advanced until it reaches the vallecula.

A straight blade is advanced over the posterior border of the epiglottis, so it is more likely to cause trauma in this area.

Left-sided blades are used in patients with right-sided facial deformities.

Polio blades were introduced in the 1950s as an aid to intubating polio sufferers in iron lungs.

They have been largely superseded by the short-handled Macintosh as used in obstetric practice.

2.115 Answers:

- A True
- B False
- C True
- D False
- E True

The letter positioning refers to: 1, chamber paced; 2, chamber sensed; 3, response to sensing; 4, programmability and rate modulation; 5, antitachyarrhythmia functions.

Hypercapnia can increase the threshold for excitation.

Older pacemakers were unipolar.

The electrode was the cathode and the box was the anode.

Newer pacemakers are bipolar.

The anode and cathode lie much closer together so reducing the risk of artefacts interrupting function.

2.116 The following should be avoided in surgical patients with modern pacemakers:

☐ A Suxamethonium

☐ B Hypothermia

☐ C Bipolar diathermy

☐ D Magnets

☐ E Nitrous oxide

2.116 Answers:

- A True
- B True
- C False
- D True
- E False

Anything causing excessive muscle movement, including fasciculation and shivering, should be avoided as it may be interpreted as cardiac muscle activity.

Bipolar diathermy can be used but unipolar diathermy should be avoided.

The routine use of magnets is no longer advocated.

Magnets were used previously to induce continuous asynchronous pacing in non-programmable pacemakers.

Currently it is thought that the effect of a magnet on the modern programmable pacemakers is unpredictable and potentially dangerous.

Pacemaker clinics are able to give information regarding response of the device to application of a magnet.

There is no reason not to use nitrous oxide.

Reference: Pacemakers and implantable cardioverter defibrillators. *Anaesthesia* 2006; 61(9): 883–90.

2.117 Surgical diathermy:

☐ A The heating power is calculated according to the product of the current squared and the resistance

☐ B The larger the tip of a surgical diathermy instrument the greater the current density

☐ C As tissue is cut, heat is dissipated to surrounding tissues

☐ D A continuous sine waveform is best for coagulation

☐ E Arcing is a method of coagulation

2.117   Answers:

- A   True
- B   False
- C   False
- D   False
- E   True

Power $= I^2 \times R$.

As tissue is cut, there is very rapid heating of tissue over a very small area.

This localised current energy results in tissue cutting without dissipation of heat to surrounding tissues.

The smaller the cutting tip, the greater the current density.

A continuous sine waveform is best for cutting.

Fulguration or spray coagulation occurs as arcing coagulates surrounding tissues.

Blunt instruments or roller balls are often used.

Reference: Surgical diathermy. *Anaesthesia and Intensive Care Medicine* 2004; 5: 369–71.

2.118 Regarding surgical diathermy:

- ☐ A Monopolar diathermy can be used only for cutting
- ☐ B Both electrodes have high current density in monopolar diathermy
- ☐ C Bipolar diathermy has high power
- ☐ D It uses radio waves
- ☐ E It operates at frequencies of 0.5–1 kHz

2.118 Answers:

- A False
- B False
- C False
- D True
- E False

Diathermy utilises alternating current at frequencies of 0.5–1 MHz.

As discussed earlier a continuous sine wave is best for cutting whereas a pulsed sine wave is best for coagulation.

Although the current density is high at the tip of the surgical instrument, it is very low at the patient plate electrode.

A low current density is achieved with a large surface area and good contact with the skin; this avoids burns.

Monopolar diathermy has higher power and is used for both cutting and coagulation.

Bipolar diathermy has low power compared with monopolar.

Reference: Surgical diathermy. *Anaesthesia and Intensive Care Medicine* 2004; 5: 369–71.

2.119 The following is true regarding diathermy smoke:

☐ A It is filtered by surgical masks

☐ B Viable HIV proviral DNA has been found in diathermy smoke

☐ C The median particle size produced is <0.5 μm in diameter

☐ D It has not been found to contain carcinogens

☐ E It contains toxins that can affect the central nervous system (CNS)

2.120 Regarding the connection between pipeline gas and the anaesthetic machine:

☐ A Piped gases terminate in theatre in a self-closing Schrader socket

☐ B A flexible hosepipe with specific diameter-indexing collar ensures the correct connection of gases

☐ C The flexible hosepipes are black reinforced rubber

☐ D Non-interchangeable screw threads (NISTs) attach the hosepipe to the anaesthetic machine

☐ E All parts of NISTs are specific to a particular gas

2.119 Answers:

- A False
- B True
- C True
- D False
- E True

Surgical masks do not filter out diathermy smoke.

They do not trap particles that are <0.5 μm in diameter.

Diathermy smoke has been found to contain proviral HIV DNA, viable bacteria and human papillomavirus DNA under experimental conditions.

The median particle size is 0.31 μm.

It has also been found to contain benzene, which is carcinogenic.

Other chemical contaminants can cause eye, skin, hepatic, renal and CNS toxicity.

Reference: Occupational hazards of anaesthesia. *Continuing Education in Anaesthesia, Critical Care and Pain* 2006; 6(5): 182–7.

2.120 Answers:

- A True
- B True
- C False
- D True
- E False

The flexible hosepipes were previously all black (reinforced rubber).

Now they are colour coded for the gas they carry.

NISTs are composed of a probe that is specific for each gas and a nut that is the same (diameter and thread) on all pipes.

The nut cannot be attached until the probe is engaged.

2.121 The following are correct regarding cylinder connection to the anaesthetic machine:

□ A They are mounted to the anaesthetic machine on yokes

□ B A pin index system exists on the yoke

□ C A Bodok sealing washer must be placed between the valve and the yoke of the anaesthetic machine

□ D Bodok seals are non-compressible

□ E The fitting between the valve block and the cylinder neck melts at low temperatures to avoid the risk of explosion

2.122 The following are correct regarding the pin index:

□ A For oxygen it is 3 and 5

□ B For nitrous oxide it is 2 and 6

□ C For air it is 1 and 6

□ D It is used only for cylinders of size E or smaller

□ E Entonox does not have a pin index

2.121 Answers:

- A True
- B True
- C True
- D False
- E True

Pins protruding from the yoke are gas cylinder specific.

A Bodok seal, which is non-combustible, compressible and composed of neoprene with aluminium edges, sits between the yoke and the cylinder head.

The cylinder neck and valve block are separated by a safety fitting that melts at low temperatures, allowing leakage of gas to reduce the risk of explosions.

Reference: Modern anaesthetic machines. Continuing education in anaesthesia, critical care and pain. *British Journal of Anaesthesia* 2006; 6(2): 75–78.

2.122 Answers:

- A False
- B False
- C False
- D False
- E False

The pin index system is used for size E cylinders and smaller.

The exception to this is the size F and G size entonox cylinders, which also have pin indexes.

The following are correct pin indexes: oxygen 2 and 5; nitrous oxide 3 and 5; air 1 and 5; and carbon dioxide 1 and 6.

2.123 Gas storage. The following are stored in cylinders in their vapour form at room temperature:

☐ A Nitrous oxide

☐ B Oxygen

☐ C Helium

☐ D Carbon dioxide

☐ E Entonox

2.124 Correct cylinder pressures at room temperature are:

☐ A Oxygen 13 700 kPa

☐ B Air 13 700 kPa

☐ C Carbon dioxide 13 700 kPa

☐ D Nitrous oxide 4400 kPa

☐ E Entonox 14 000 kPa

2.123 Answers:

- A   True
- B   False
- C   False
- D   True
- E   False

Remember a gas exists in its gaseous state at room temperature if its critical temperature ie the temperature above which it cannot be liquefied by pressure alone, is below room temperature.

Its critical temperature, ie the temperature above which it cannot be liquefied by pressure alone, so is below room temperature, it cannot be liquefied; therefore it is stored as a gas.

A vapour is a substance in its gaseous form beneath its critical temperature.

Both carbon dioxide and nitrous oxide exist as vapours at room temperature.

The critical temperature for nitrous oxide is 36.5°C and the critical temperature for carbon dioxide is 31°C.

2.124 Answers:

- A   True
- B   True
- C   False
- D   True
- E   False

At room temperature air and oxygen have a cylinder pressure of 13 700 kPa.

Entonox is stored as a gas at room temperature at 13 700 kPa.

Carbon dioxide is stored as a liquid at room temperature at a pressure of 50 bars.

It has a critical temperature of 31°C.

Nitrous oxide is stored as a liquid at room temperature at 44 bars.

1 bar = 101.325 kPa

2.125 Storage of oxygen. Vacuum insulated evaporators (VIEs):

☐ A   Can be housed on hospital sites

☐ B   Contain liquid oxygen stored at temperatures above −150°C

☐ C   Contain liquid oxygen stored at 4 bars

☐ D   Can be weighed to determine the amount of stored oxygen

☐ E   Are routinely fitted with a safety valve opening at 17 bars

2.126 Oxygen concentrators:

☐ A   Extract oxygen from air

☐ B   Can be designed to provide oxygen for single patient use at home

☐ C   Comprise hydrated aluminium silicate columns

☐ D   Achieve a maximum oxygen concentration of 97%

☐ E   Argon is the main remaining constituent

2.125 Answers:

- A True
- B False
- C False
- D True
- E True

VIEs are economical for storage and supply of oxygen.

Oxygen is stored in liquid form, ie beneath its critical temperature of −118°C.

It is kept at temperatures of approximately −160°C and at pressures of 5–10 bars and is fitted with a safety pressure-reducing value if the pressure exceeds 17 bars.

As oxygen is used and gas pressure falls liquid oxygen is taken from the bottom of the vessel and passed through a superheater (insulated coils of copper) to return the oxygen pressure to the required levels.

2.126 Answers:

- A True
- B True
- C True
- D False
- E True

Oxygen concentrators can be used to supply single patient use or to supply oxygen for pipeline systems.

The functioning unit is a zeolite (hydrated aluminium silicate) molecular sieve, which separates oxygen from nitrogen.

Air is compressed and cooled, then exposed to the sieve where it is dried and oxygen is separated off.

The maximum oxygen concentration achieved is 90–95%, with 2–5% argon remaining as a contaminant.

2.127   Regarding entonox:

☐ A   It is a 50 : 50 mixture of oxygen and nitrous oxide

☐ B   Mixture can exhibit the Poynting effect at temperatures below its pseudo-critical temperature

☐ C   The Poynting effect is most marked if the cylinder pressure before cooling is 117 bars

☐ D   Prolonged use can precipitate haemolytic anaemia

☐ E   High cylinder temperatures can present an increased risk of delivering a hypoxic mixture

2.128   Medical air:

☐ A   Is routinely supplied at two different pressures: 4 bars and 7 bars

☐ B   At high pressure is often used to drive operating tools

☐ C   In cylinders has a PIN (pin index number) of 1 and 6

☐ D   In cylinders is black with black and white shoulders

☐ E   In cylinders is stored at 4 bars

2.127 Answers:

- A True
- B True
- C True
- D False
- E False

Entonox is a 50 : 50 oxygen : nitrous oxide mix.

At temperatures below pseudo-critical temperature (−5.5°C) the mixture is prone to liquefaction and separation, which can lead to delivery of hypoxic mix (once the oxygen has been used).

Prolonged use can cause bone marrow depression but not haemolytic anaemia.

At 117 bars the mixture is most prone to separation.

Increasing or decreasing the temperature decreases the risk of separation.

2.128 Answers:

- A True
- B True
- C False
- D False
- E False

Medical air is used to power many operating tools at pressures of 700 kPa or 7 bars.

It has a PIN of 1 and 5 and is in grey cylinders with black and white shoulders.

Cylinder pressure is 137 bars or 13 700 kPa.

2.129 Regarding pressure gauges:

☐ A Cylinder pressures are measured with aneroid gauges

☐ B The cross-section of the coiled tube in a Bourdon gauge is circular in shape

☐ C The inner end of the tube within a Bourdon gauge is sealed

☐ D A needle pointer is used as an indicator of pressure on a calibrated gauge

☐ E The face of a pressure gauge is made of non-specific but clear glass

2.130 Flow meters:

☐ A Are constant orifice, variable pressure meters

☐ B At low flows are governed by viscosity of the gas

☐ C At low flows obey laws of laminar flow

☐ D Are calibrated for specific gases

☐ E At high flows are determined by the density of the gas

2.129 Answers:

- A True
- B False
- C True
- D True
- E False

Bourdon gauges or aneroid gauges are used to measure cylinder and pipeline pressures.

They consist of a coil of oval-shaped tubing with the outer end connected to the gas supply and a sealed inner tube connected to a needle pointer.

The face of the pressure gauge is made of reinforced heavy glass as a safety feature if the tube ruptures.

2.130 Answers:

- A False
- B True
- C True
- D True
- E True

Flow meters are gas specific.

The clearance between the bobbin and the tube wall widens as the flow of gas increases.

At low flows, the clearance is longer and narrower and therefore acts as a tube.

Flow is laminar and obeys the laws of the Hagen–Poiseuille equation and is dependant on the viscosity of the gas.

Flow = $Pd^4\pi \div 128\eta l$

At high flows, the clearance is shorter and wider and acts as an orifice.

The flow is turbulent and dependent on the density of gas.

2.131 Regarding flow meters:

- ☐ A The reading is taken from the dot in the centre of the bobbin
- ☐ B When a ball is used as a bobbin the reading is taken from the mid- point of the ball
- ☐ C They are accurate with an error margin of ±2.5%
- ☐ D Carbon dioxide and nitrous oxide have very similar properties and can therefore be used in the same flow meter
- ☐ E Oxygen is the first of the gases to be added to the mixture

2.132 Regarding vaporisers:

- ☐ A The Goldman vaporiser is an example of a vaporiser used inside the breathing circuit
- ☐ B Vaporisers inside the circle are of low resistance
- ☐ C In the Tec Mark 3 vaporiser, the bi-metallic strip controlling the splitting ratio is situated within the vaporising chamber
- ☐ D The interlocking Selecta Tec system is compatible with Tec Mark 5 and above
- ☐ E The specific heat capacity of copper is 0.39 J/g per K

2.131 Answers:

- A False
- B True
- C True
- D True
- E False

Flow meters can be made inaccurate by a number of causes including dirt, static, inaccurate calibration and the gas used.

The bobbin has a white dot to show that it is spinning and the reading is taken from the top of the bobbin or the centre of a ball.

Oxygen is added to the mixture last.

2.132 Answers:

- A True
- B True
- C False
- D False
- E True

Vaporisers can be grouped into those used within the circle or those outside the circle.

The Goldman and Oxford Miniature vaporisers are examples of those used within the circle.

Plenum vaporisers are those used outside the circle, including the Tec vaporisers.

Vaporisers within the circle must be low resistance.

Tec Mark 3–5 vaporisers have the bi-metallic strip outside the vaporising chamber.

The interlock Selecta Tec system is compatible for Tec Mark 4 and 5.

Copper readily gives its heat to the gas within the vaporiser so maintaining the temperature of the anaesthetic gas.

2.133 Regarding vaporisers:

☐ A Isoflurane in vaporisers contains a preservative

☐ B A pressure relief valve downstream of the vaporiser opens at 45 kPa

☐ C Minute volume divider ventilators exert backpressure on vaporisers as they cycle

☐ D Tec Mark 3 has a long outlet port to avoid contamination by retrograde flow

☐ E The specific heat capacity of the copper sink of a vaporiser is greater than that of water

2.134 Regarding ventilators:

☐ A Pressure-triggered ventilators decrease the work of breathing when compared with flow-triggered ventilators

☐ B Time cycling is used in pressure-controlled ventilation

☐ C Flow cycling is used in pressure-supported ventilation

☐ D Volume cycling is used in volume-controlled ventilation

☐ E In pressure-controlled ventilators, the flow decelerates through the breath to maintain the targeted pressure at the peak of inspired pressure

2.133 Answers:

- A False
- B False
- C True
- D False
- E False

Halothane vaporisers contain the preservative thymol but enflurane and isoflurane do not contain preservatives.

The pressure relief valve serves to protect the machinery, not the patient.

It releases at pressures of 35 kPa.

Other safety features to protect against backpressure causing contamination include downstream flow resistors and equal capacity in the bypass channel and the vaporising chamber.

The specific heat capacity of copper is 0.39 J/g per K compared with that of water at 4.18 J/g per K.

The Tec Mk3 has a long inlet port to prevent contamination.

2.134 Answers:

- A False
- B True
- C True
- D True
- E True

Flow-triggered ventilators reduce the work of breathing compared with pressure-triggered ventilators because there is always some background gas flow for the patient and no delay in inspiratory valve opening.

Flow cycling used in pressure-supported ventilation cycles the ventilator into expiration when there is a reduction of the peak inspired flow.

Volume-cycling ventilators begin expiration once a set tidal volume has been delivered.

2.135 Servo ventilators:

☐ A Operate by bag-in-bottle technique

☐ B Are used with a circle breathing system

☐ C Rely on pneumotachography to activate inspiratory and expiratory flow

☐ D Are driven by oxygen

☐ E Are minute volume dividers

2.136 Regarding double-lumen tubes:

☐ A They were initially derived from Carlen's tube

☐ B Robertshaw tubes are better designed to avoid right upper lobe collapse compared with the bronchocath

☐ C Robertshaw tubes are sized as per French gauge

☐ D It is better to use a right-sided tube for right-sided thoracic surgery

☐ E Open pleurectomy is an absolute indication for endobronchial intubation

2.135 Answers:

- A False
- B False
- C True
- D False
- E True

Servo ventilators are minute volume dividers.

A bag is filled with gas from the fresh gas flow.

A spring compresses the bag and pushes gas into the inspiratory limb.

Flow is measured with a pneumotachograph.

Once the divided volume has been delivered, the inspiratory limb is clamped and the expiratory limb opens.

The expiratory limb is vented to scavenging and so not returned to the patient as in a circle system.

2.136 Answers:

- A True
- B True
- C False
- D False
- E False

Carlens' tube was introduced in 1949 to allow measurement of individual lung volumes.

Robertshaw tubes are the classic red rubber tubes.

They are better designed to avoid right upper lobe obstruction and collapse as their slot is almost two times the length of the equivalent bronchocath.

Bronchocaths are French gauge sizes 35, 37, 39, 41 and 28 left.

Robertshaw tubes are extra small, small, medium or large.

A left-sided tube is best for right thoracic surgery as it allows decompression of the right lung and left lung ventilation.

Open pleurectomy is a relative indication for using a double-lumen tube.

2.137 Regarding soda lime:

☐ A One kilogram can absorb 120 litres of carbon dioxide

☐ B It consists of granule size 4–8 mesh

☐ C It should be shaped as uniformed spheres 3–4 mm in diameter

☐ D It consists of predominantly calcium hydroxide

☐ E With smaller particle size it offers less resistance to flow

2.137   Answers:

- A   True
- B   True
- C   True
- D   True
- E   False

Here 4–8 mesh describes granules of the size that will fit through strainers with 4–8 openings per inch (2.5 cm).

Smaller granules offer less resistance to flow and the dust caused by very small particles can be caustic.

The uniform spheres of 3–4 mm shape reduce channelling and allow a more even flow of gases.

The inter-granular space in soda lime should approximate to the patient's tidal volume.

Statistics

MCQs

Indicate your answers with a tick or cross in the boxes provided.

2.138 The following are examples of ordinal data:

☐ A ASA grade

☐ B Age

☐ C GCS grade

☐ D Weight

☐ E Blood group

2.138 Answers:

- A True
- B False
- C True
- D False
- E False

Ordinal data are ranked data.

Each subject is allocated to a mutually exclusive group but the groups have an intrinsic ranking.

They are not, however, part of a scale, eg ASA grade 4 is not twice as bad as ASA grade 2.

Nominal data are not ranked and bear no numerical relationship to each other, eg sex or blood group.

Numerical data can be either discrete or continuous.

Discrete data can take only certain values, eg number of sisters.

Continuous data can take any numerical value, eg height, weight or blood pressure.

Reference: Statistics. *Anaesthesia and Intensive Care Medicine* 2002; 3: 428–33.

2.139 Regarding a box-and-whisker plot:

☐ A The vertical line represents the range

☐ B The horizontal line represents the mean

☐ C The box represents the percentiles

☐ D An asterisk signifies an outlier

☐ E It is useful for demonstrating the mode

2.139 Answers:

- A True
- B False
- C True
- D True
- E False

Box-and-whisker plots are helpful in interpreting the distribution of data.

The vertical line represents range, the horizontal line represents the median, the box represents percentiles (commonly the 2.5th to the 97.5th).

Sometimes one piece of the data falls well outside the range of the other values.

This piece of the data is known as an outlier.

So as not to give the impression that the results are dispersed throughout the range, this is not included in the plot and an asterisk is shown.

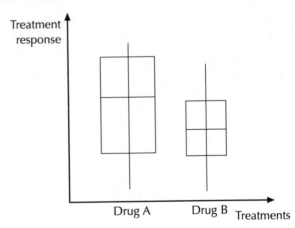

Figure: Box-and-whisker plot

Reference: Statistics. *Anaesthesia and Intensive Care Medicine* 2002; 3: 428–33.

2.140 The following statistical statements are correct:

☐ A In normal distribution, mean = mode = median

☐ B In normal distribution, the variability is described by the standard deviation

☐ C The mean is the best indicator of central location in skewed data

☐ D Standard deviation of a sample that is more than half the mean is likely to be skewed data

☐ E The mean is a good measure of central location in continuously variable data

2.141 Standard error of the mean (SEM):

☐ A Is the standard deviation of the sampling distribution of the mean

☐ B Is calculated by the formula: standard deviation of the original distribution × sample size

☐ C Is calculated by a formula that assumes that the original or true population data are normally distributed

☐ D Is used to calculate the 95% confidence interval for the true population using the following equation: sample mean ± 2× SEM)

☐ E Decreases as the likelihood of it representing the true population increases

2.140   Answers:

- A   True
- B   True
- C   False
- D   True
- E   True

In skewed data, if the single largest result is much increased this will affect the mean, but will have no effect on the median or mode and therefore they are better indicators of central position.

The mean is a good indicator of central location in continuously variable data; however mode and median are better indicators in ordinal and numerical data.

Reference: Statistics. *Anaesthesia and Intensive Care Medicine* 2002; 3: 428–33.

2.141   Answers:

- A   True
- B   False
- C   False
- D   True
- E   True

The standard error of the mean is inferential statistics.

One inference is that, if several samples are taken from a population (not necessarily normally distributed) and their means are plotted, they will form a normal distribution around the true population mean.

The SEM is the standard deviation of these sample means.

The SEM is calculated by the formula: standard deviation of the sample/square root of sample numbers.

As the sample size increases, the SEM decreases, ie the sample mean is more closely related to the true population mean.

Reference: Statistics. *Anaesthesia and Intensive Care Medicine* 2002; 3: 428–33.

2.142 Regarding statistics:

☐ A Non-parametric tests make no assumption regarding the underlying distribution of the data

☐ B Parametric tests can be used for all data interpretation

☐ C In normally distributed data, 1.96 standard deviations on either side of the mean encompass 95% of the population

☐ D A null hypothesis assumes that there is no difference between analysed groups

☐ E Type 1 error occurs when there is a difference in treatments but the study fails to identify it

2.142 Answers:

- A True
- B False
- C True
- D True
- E False

Statistical techniques that make no assumption of the underlying distribution of the data are non-parametric.

These tests can be used on any type of data.

Parametric tests assume that the data are normally distributed.

However, provided that the data are continuously variable with deviations that are not too extreme, even non-normal distributions can be safely analysed.

A type 1 error occurs when the null hypothesis is rejected, ie a difference between groups is identified but there is actually no difference.

This is expected in 5% of cases when a *P* value <0.05 is accepted.

A type 2 error is more common.

This results from an acceptance of the null hypothesis, ie not identifying a difference between the groups when a difference actually exists.

The commonest cause for this is small sample size.

2.143 The following are appropriate tests for statistical analysis:

- ☐ A Contingency tables for categorical data
- ☐ B Unpaired Mann–Whitney test for ordinal data
- ☐ C Friedman's test for categorical data
- ☐ D Unpaired *t*-test for continuously variable data normally distributed
- ☐ E Analysis of variance for ordinal data

2.143 Answers:

- A True
- B True
- C False
- D True
- E False

The chart below shows the appropriate tests for the collected data.

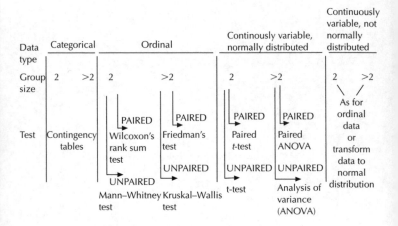

Figure: Collected data tests

2.144 Linear regression: regarding $y = mx + c$:

☐ A It is the equation for a straight line

☐ B y is the independent variable

☐ C m is the slope of the line

☐ D c intercepts the line on the x axis

☐ E A scattergram helps to confirm that the data are appropriated for linear analysis

2.144 Answers:

- A True
- B False
- C True
- D False
- E True

$y = mx + c$ where y is the dependent variable, x is the independent variable, m is the slope of the line and c is the point of intercept with the y axis.

This is the equation for a straight line.

It is for analysis of the amount of change of one variable caused by another.

It compares two parametric variables for association.

A scattergram should be plotted and displayed in the literature to check for obvious deviations in the data and other patterns in the data that could be missed by computer analysis.

Reference: Statistics: Part 2. *Anaesthesia and Intensive Care Medicine* 2003; 4: 203–6.

2.145 Regarding correlation statistics:

☐ A Correlation measures the degree of linear association of two independent variables

☐ B If two variables are correlated the relationship must be causal

☐ C A Pearson correlation coefficient r of -1 signifies that both variables increase together

☐ D The value r^2 is the coefficient of determination

☐ E Spearman's rank correlation coefficient is used for parametric data

2.145 Answers:

- A True
- B False
- C False
- D True
- E False

The Pearson correlation coefficient is used for parametric data analysis and indicates the degree of association only.

$r = +1$ signifies a positive relationship, ie both variables increase together.

$r = -1$ signifies an inverse relationship, ie one increases as the other decreases.

Both $r = +1$ and $r = -1$ will yield a straight line.

As the scatter around the line of best fit increases, r approaches 0.

The coefficient of determination is r^2, which measures the change of one variable that is associated with change in the other.

$1 - r^2$ is the amount of change of one variable that is unrelated to the other variable, ie is due to other factors.

The Spearman rank correlation coefficient is used for the examination of relationship between ordinal data.

Reference: Statistics: Part 2. *Anaesthesia and Intensive Care Medicine* 2003; 4: 203–6.

2.146 Regarding statistics:

☐ A Meta-analysis can be easily biased

☐ B Number needed to treat (NNT) is the reciprocal of the absolute risk reduction of a treatment

☐ C A β-error of 10% will mean that a study has a 90% chance of detecting a difference between groups, should a difference exist

☐ D The sensitivity of a test is defined as the true positives divided by the sum of the true positives and the false negatives.

☐ E The accuracy of a test is defined as the true positives divided by the sum of the true positives and the false positives

2.146 Answers:

- A True
- B True
- C True
- D True
- E False

Meta-analysis must be interpreted with caution.

The sample selection must be unbiased, otherwise the results of the meta-analysis will be inaccurate as in the case of the meta-analysis of intravenous magnesium in reduction of risk of mortality post-myocardial infarction.

Studies may not be published if they do not show a positive benefit.

If only published studies are incorporated in the meta-analysis, the data will be positively biased.

A central register of all clinical trials would reduce this bias.

The author's selection of trials for the meta-analysis can add significant bias.

A single randomised control trial can strongly influence the overall result in certain circumstances.

The NNT is the number in the group that would need to receive treatment in order for one participant to have the desired effect.

A β-error is a type II error, ie rejection of a result as being due to chance when there is a real difference.

A value of 20% is usually considered the maximum acceptable.

Option E refers to the positive predictive value.

The accuracy of a test is defined as the sum of the true positives and the true negatives divided by the total.

2.147 The following are true regarding a *P* value < 0.001:

☐ A   It implies great statistical significance

☐ B   It implies clinical significance

☐ C   If the test were performed 100 times, only once would it reveal
a positive result by chance

☐ D   It represents the α-error

☐ E   It represents the power of the study

2.147 Answers:

- A True
- B False
- C False
- D True
- E False

A *P* value is statistically significant if it is less than 0.05.

Statistical significance does not necessarily imply clinical significance.

A *P* value of 0.001 implies that, if the test were performed 1000 times, only once would it reveal a positive result by chance.

A type I error or an α-error is a false positive, ie a finding that a result is positive and significant when in fact it occurred by chance.

The power of a study is $(1 - \beta)$ or $(1 - \text{type II error})$.

Where a type II error is a false negative, ie the result is positive but is rejected as it is thought to be caused by chance.

2.148 Non-parametric tests:

☐ A Can be used to assess ordinal data

☐ B Include Fisher's exact test

☐ C Can be used to assess the difference in sex between groups

☐ D Include Student *t*-tests

☐ E Cannot be used to assess data where the distribution is unknown

2.149 Regarding normal distribution:

☐ A The variance is synonymous with the mean

☐ B 10% of the population will fall outside $2 \times$ SD from the mean

☐ C The standard deviation represents the variability of the sample

☐ D The mode is the same as the median

☐ E Analysis of variance is a statistical test designed to analyse this type of data

2.148 Answers:

- A True
- B True
- C True
- D False
- E False

Non-parametric tests are used to assess data that are not normally distributed or that have an unknown distribution.

Non-parametric tests include χ^2 tests or Fisher's exact test (if any expected frequency < 5), for nominal data and Mann–Whitney rank sum test or Kruskal–Wallis for ordinal data.

Examples of parametric tests include Student's *t*-test, analysis of variance and paired *t*-tests.

Difference in sex is an example of nominal data and can be assessed using non-parametric tests.

2.149 Answers:

- A False
- B False
- C True
- D True
- E True

In normally distributed data, mean = mode = median.

The square root of the variance is the standard deviation, which represents the variability of the sample.

The mean ± 1 SD contains 67% of the observations.

The mean ± 2 SD contains 95% of the observations.

The mean ± 3 SD contains 99% of the observations.

2.150 Regarding basic measurement concepts:

☐   A   Gradient drift is corrected with a single point calibration

☐   B   Temperature changes in a blood pressure transducer can be a cause of drift

☐   C   Offset drift varies by the same amount per period

☐   D   Linearity is calculated according to the relationship of the true to the displayed value

☐   E   Transducers used in clinical practice usually have a non-linearity less than 1%

2.150 Answers:

- A False
- B True
- C True
- D True
- E True

Drift occurs when, over a period, the displayed value differs from the true value.

Offset drift occurs when the displayed value varies by a constant from the true value; this can be corrected by a single point calibration.

Gradient drift occurs when the displayed value varies from the true value by different amounts at different times.

Gradient drift develops less rapidly than offset drift.

A two-point calibration is required for its correction.

Linearity is calculated according to the relationship of the true to the displayed value.

A proportionality constant is generated.

When displayed value is always equal to the true value, this constant is 1.

CORE TEXT REFERENCES

Baha Al-Shaikh, Stacy S. *Essentials of Anaesthetic Equipment.* 2nd edn. Churchill Livingstone 2001.

Davis PD, Parbrook GD, *Basic Physics and Measurement in Anaesthesia.* 4th edn. Butterworth-Heinemann 1995.

Davis PD, Kenny G. *Basic Physics and Measurement in Anaesthesia.* 5th edn. Butterworth-Heinemann 2001.

Yentis, Hirsch, Smith. *Anaesthesia and Intensive Care A–Z. An encyclopaedia of principles and practice* 3rd edn. Butterworth-Heinemann 2004.

INDEX

Locators in bold refer to book number, those in normal type refer to question number.

Index

index

214

Index

Index

Index

Index

221

Index